A PRACTICAL GUIDE TO ULTRASOUND
OF FETAL ANOMALIES

A Practical Guide to Ultrasound of Fetal Anomalies

Frederick N. Hegge, M.D.
Director, Ultrasound Department
Emanuel Hospital
Portland, Oregon

Raven Press **New York**

Raven Press Ltd., 1185 Avenue of the Americas, New York, New York 10036

Made in the United States of America

Library of Congress Cataloging-in-Publication Data

Hegge, Frederick N.
    A practical guide to ultrasound of fetal anomalies / Frederick N.
  Hegge.
        p.   cm.
    Includes index.
    ISBN 0-88167-845-7 (pbk.)
    1. Fetus—Abnormalities—Ultrasonic imaging.   I. Title.
    [DNLM: 1. Abnormalities—diagnosis. 2. Fetal Diseases—diagnosis.
    3. Ultrasonography, Prenatal—methods. WQ 211 H463p]
  RG628.3.U58H45   1991
  618.3'207543—dc20
  DNLM/DLC
  for Library of Congress   91-28787
                                                                        CIP

The material contained in this volume was submitted as previously unpublished material, except in the instances in which credit has been given to the source from which some of the illustrative material was derived.

Great care has been taken to maintain the accuracy of the information contained in the volume. However, neither Raven Press nor the editors can be held responsible for errors or for any consequences arising from the use of the information contained herein.

9 8 7 6 5 4 3 2 1

Contents

Preface

"In the fields of observation, chance favors only the mind that is prepared."

Louis Pasteur

A Practical Guide to Ultrasound of Fetal Anomalies is intended for sonographers and sonologists in training and for those in practice who perform basic obstetric ultrasound. Chapters 1–3 of Section I briefly review background information about congenital anomalies. In Chapters 4 through 8 an approach to the fetal anatomy survey is presented that is designed to meet emerging standards of practice in a practical and effective manner. Section II presents an atlas that contains numerous examples of the anomalies sought by the fetal anatomy survey.

Much of the book is based on the classification of fetal anomalies according to the steps of the fetal anatomy survey. This approach lessens the difficulty of learning the large number of detectable anomalies by presenting each part of the fetal anatomy survey as an active search for a smaller and more manageable group of specific anomalies.

The extensive atlas of Section II prepares the reader to recognize the anomalies that are sought. This atlas enhances the learning process by presenting numerous examples of anomalies in chapters organized according to the fetal anatomy survey. This organization of the atlas makes this book an easy-to-use reference when possible abnormalities are encountered during the fetal anatomy survey.

Frederick N. Hegge, M.D.

Acknowledgments

I would like to thank Emanuel Hospital for its generous support. Thanks especially to Emanuel Hospital photographer David Lawton for his diligence in reproducing the many images shown in the book. I would also like to thank Dr. Michael J. Daly and Dr. Douglas H. King for reviewing portions of the manuscript.

Frederick N. Hegge, M.D.

SECTION I

Congenital Anomalies and the Fetal Anatomy Survey

Chapter 1

CONGENITAL ANOMALIES

Children are considered to have congenital anomalies when they have structural defects at or soon after birth, including tumors and syndromes that are likely to be associated with structural defects (1). This definition includes malformations occurring during embryogenesis, such as neural tube defects, as well as disruptions of fetal development occurring later in gestation, such as porencephaly after fetal cerebral hemorrhage. Only 60% of congenital anomalies are obvious at birth (2).

A large multicenter study conducted in the 1960s found that 6.5% of children have major or minor congenital anomalies, 0.4% have syndromes, and 0.3% have tumors (Table 1.1). Because some children have multiple anomalies, as many as 8.8 anomalies per 100 children are present (1).

Major anomalies are defined as being life threatening, requiring major surgery, or having serious cosmetic effects. Minor anomalies do not meet these criteria. Major anomalies are present in 3.2% of children, and minor anomalies are present in 3.6% (Tables 1.2, 1.3). The total of the two groups exceeds the 6.5% total for all children with anomalies because of slight overlap. Minor anomalies considered to be trivial, such as cleft uvula, are not included in these totals (1).

Major congenital anomalies are an important cause of pregnancy wastage and infant mortality and morbidity. They are found in more than one-half of all spontaneous abortuses and approximately 20% of all stillborn fetuses, and they are associated with 15% of neonatal deaths. In addition, major anomalies are a common cause of hospitalization or death in early childhood (2).

TABLE 1.1. *Percentages of children who have congenital anomalies*[a]

Any anomaly	6.5%
Major	3.2%
Minor	3.6%
Syndromes	0.4%
Tumors	0.3%

[a] When children with multiple anomalies are considered, the occurrence rate of anomalies is 8.8 per 100 children (1).

TABLE 1.2. *Rate of major congenital anomalies per 100 children (1)*

Central nervous	0.69
Cardiovascular	1.04
Musculoskeletal	0.75
Respiratory	0.36
Gastrointestinal	0.43
Genitourinary	0.62
Eye and ear	0.17
	4.06

TABLE 1.3. *Rate of minor congenital anomalies per 100 children (1)*

Hernias (inguinal, umbilical, etc.)	1.5
Polydactyly (isolated)	0.7
Hypospadias	0.4
Cleft gum	0.2
Pectus excavatum	0.2
Urethral obstruction	0.1
Vertebrae, ribs, sternum, hands, feet	0.1
Abnormal lung lobulation	0.1
Preauricular skin tag	0.1
Other	0.4
	3.8

TABLE 1.4. *Selected factors found to increase the risk of fetal anomalies in a large multicenter study[a]*

	Relative risk
Single umbilical artery	4.1
Low birth weight (less than 1,500 gm)	3.1
Malformed siblings (three or more)	2.9
Polyhydramnios	2.4
Treated maternal diabetes (five years)	2.4
Convulsive disorder	1.7
Maternal coagulation defect	1.7
Hemorrhagic shock during pregnancy	1.6
Maternal age greater than 40 years	1.5
Maternal age less than 14 years	1.4

[a] Modified from ref. 1.

TABLE 1.5. *Rates of chromosome abnormalities per 100 live births for selected maternal ages[a]*

Maternal age	(Down) Trisomy 21	(Edwards) Trisomy 18	(Patu) Trisomy 13	XXY	Other (XYY, XO, etc.)	Total
15	0.10	<0.01	<0.01	0.04	0.08	0.22
20	0.06	<0.01	<0.01	0.04	0.08	0.19
25	0.08	0.01	<0.01	0.04	0.08	0.21
30	0.11	0.02	<0.02	0.05	0.08	0.26
35	0.32	0.04	0.03	0.09	0.09	0.56
40	1.11	0.13	0.08	0.18	0.09	1.58
45	4.05	0.44	0.28	0.51	0.09	5.37
49	11.43	1.26	0.78	1.38	0.09	14.93

[a] Modified table reprinted from ref. 3 with permission of The American College of Obstetricians and Gynecologists.

Many risk factors are known to increase significantly the likelihood of congenital anomalies over the background rate that already seems rather high. The previously cited multicenter study documents the association of congenital anomalies with many factors, including single umbilical artery, low birth weight, anomalous siblings, polyhydramnios, maternal diabetes, and very young or advanced maternal age (Table 1.4) (1).

Other studies document the importance of additional maternal risk factors, including age-related tendency to chromosomal abnormalities, exposure to chemicals or drugs, and infection with toxoplasma, varicella, rubella, herpes, cytomegalovirus, or syphilis (Tables 1.5, 1.6, and 1.7) (3–7). Hereditary syndromes and other syndromes too numerous for tabulation are discussed in more comprehensive reference books (5–7). A few highly selected examples of syndromes are listed in Table 1.8.

TABLE 1.6. *Congenital anomalies associated with congenital infection (6,7)*

	CMV	Toxo	Ru	Syph	HS	Var
Microcephaly	X	X	X	X	X	
Hydrocephaly	X	X	X	X		
Hydranencephaly					X	
Dandy-Walker	X	X	X			
Periventricular calcif.	X	X				
Cardiac abnormality			X			
Liver calcif.	X					X
Extremity abnormality						X
Other	X	X	X	X	X	X

CMV, cytomegalovirus; Toxo, toxoplasma; Ru, rubella; Syph, syphilis; HS, herpes simplex; Var, varicella. Sonographically detectable anomalies are emphasized (5–7).

TABLE 1.7. *Common drugs and chemicals described in association with sonographically detectable fetal anomalies (not all are proven to be teratogenic)[a]*

Drug	Fetal abnormalities
Acetaminophen	Polyhydramnios
Acetazolamide	Sacrococcygeal teratoma
Acetylsalicylic acid	Intracranial hemorrhage, growth retardation
Albuterol	Fetal tachycardia
Alcohol	Microcephaly, short nose, hypoplastic maxilla, micrognathia, skeletal abnormalities, growth retardation
Amantadine	Single ventricle with pulmonary atresia
Aminopterin	Meningoencephalocele, hydrocephalus, incomplete skull ossification, brachycephaly, anencephaly, hypoplasia of thumb and fibula, clubfoot, syndactyly, hypognathia
Amitriptyline	Micrognathia, limb reduction, swelling of hands and feet, urinary retention
Amobarbital	Anencephaly, heart defects, severe limb deformities, hip dislocation, polydactyly, clubfoot, oral cleft, intersex, soft tissue deformity of neck
Antithyroid drugs	Goiter
Azathioprine	Pulmonary valvular stenosis, polydactyly
Betamethasone	Reduced head circumference
Bromides	Polydactyly, clubfoot, hip dislocation
Busulfan	Pyloric stenosis, cleft palate, microphthalmia, growth retardation
Caffeine	Musculoskeletal defects, hydronephrosis
Captopril	Leg reduction
Carbon monoxide	Cerebral atrophy, hydrocephalus, stillbirth
Carbamazepine	Meningomyelocele, atrial septal defect, patent ductus arteriosus, nose hypoplasia, hypertelorism, hip dislocation, cleft lip
Chlordiazepoxide	Microcephaly, heart defects, duodenal atresia
Chloroquine	Hemihypertrophy
Chlorpheniramine	Hydrocephalus, polydactyly, hip dislocation
Chlorpropamide	Microcephaly, dysmorphic hands and fingers
Clomiphene	Meningomyelocele, hydrocephalus, microcephaly, anencephaly, syndactyly, clubfoot, polydactyly, esophageal atresia
Codeine	Hydrocephalus, heart defects, musculoskeletal defects, hip dislocation, pyloric stenosis, oral cleft, respiratory malformations
Cortisone	Hydrocephalus, ventricular septal defect, coarctation of aorta, clubfoot, cleft lip
Coumadin	Encephalocele, anencephaly, spina bifida, heart defects, nasal hypoplasia, scoliosis, skeletal deformities, stippled epiphysis, chondroplasia punctata, short phalanges, toe defects, incomplete rotation of gut, growth retardation, bleeding
Cyclophosphamide	Tetralogy of Fallot, flattened nasal bridge, four toes on each foot, hypoplastic mid phalanx, syndactyly

TABLE 1.7. *Continued*

Drug	Fetal abnormalities
Cytarabine	Anencephaly, tetralogy of Fallot, lobster claw of three digits, missing feet digits, syndactyly
Daunorubicin	Anencephaly, tetralogy of Fallot, syndactyly, growth retardation
Dextroamphetamine	Exencephaly, atrial septal defect, other heart defects
Diazepam	Spina bifida, heart defects, absence of arm, syndactyly, absence of thumbs, cleft lip/palate
Diphenhydramine	Clubfoot, cleft palate
Disulfiram	Vertebral fusion, clubfoot, radial aplasia, phocomelia, tracheoesophageal fistula
Diuretics	Respiratory malformations
Estrogens	Heart defects, limb reduction
Ethanol	Vetricular septal defect, atrial septal defect, double outlet right ventricle, pulmonary atresia, dextrocardia, patent ductus arteriosus, tetralogy of Fallot, short nose, hypoplastic philtrum, micrognathia, pectus excavatum, radioulnar synostosis, bifid xiphoid, scoliosis, oral cleft, growth retardation, diaphragmatic hernia
Ethosuximide	Hydrocephalus, short neck, oral cleft
Fluorouracil	Radial aplasia, absent thumbs, aplasia of esophagus and duodenum, hypoplasia of lungs
Fluphenazine	Poor ossification of frontal bone, oral cleft
Haloperidol	Limb deformities
Heparin	Bleeding
Progestogenic hormones	Anencephaly, hydrocephalus, tetralogy of Fallot, truncus arteriosus, ventricular septal defect, spina bifida, absence of thumbs
Imipramine	Exencephaly, limb reduction, cleft palate, renal cystic degeneration, diaphragmatic hernia
Indomethacin	Phocomelia, stillbirth, hemorrhage
Isoniazid	Meningomyelocele
Lithium	Hydrocephalus, meningomyelocele, ventricular septal defect, Ebstein's anomaly, mitral atresia, patent ductus arteriosus, dextrocardia, spina bifida
Lysergic acid diethylamide	Hydrocephalus, encephalocele, meningomyelocele, limb deficiencies
Meclizine	Hypoplastic left heart, respiratory defects
Meprobamate	Heart defects, bilateral limb defects
Methotrexate	Oxycephaly, absence of frontal bone, large fontanelles, dextrocardia, hypoplastic mandible, long webbed fingers, growth retardation, low-set ears
Methyl mercury	Microcephaly, asymmetric head
Metronidazole	Midline facial defects
Nortriptyline	Limb reduction
Oral contraceptives	Meningomyelocele, hydrocephalus, anencephaly, heart defects, vertebral malformations, limb reduction, tracheoesophageal malformations, growth retardation

(*continued*)

TABLE 1.7. *Continued*

Drug	Fetal abnormalities
Paramethadione	Tetralogy of Fallot, growth retardation
Penicillamine	Ventricular septal defect, pyloric stenosis, growth retardation
Phenobarbital	Hydrocephalus, meningomyelocele, digital anomalies, cleft palate, ileal atresia, growth retardation, pulmonary hypoplasia
Phenothiazines	Microcephaly, syndactyly, clubfoot, omphalocele, abdominal distention
Phenylephrine	Eye and ear abnormalities, syndactyly, clubfoot, hip dislocation, umbilical hernia
Phenylpropanolamine	Pectus excavatum, polydactyly, hip dislocation
Phenytoin	Microcephaly, heart defects, rib/sternal abnormalities, short nose, broad nasal bridge, wide fontanelles, broad alveolar ridge, short neck, hypertelorism, low-set ears, hypoplastic distal phalanges, digital thumb, hip dislocation, cleft palate/lip, growth retardation
Polychlorinated biphenyls	Spotted calcification in skull, fontanelle and sagittal suture, stillbirth, growth retardation
Primidone	Ventricular septal defect, webbed neck, small mandible
Procarbazine	Cerebral hemorrhage, oligodactyly
Quinine	Hydrocephalus, heart defects, facial defects, vertebral anomalies, dysmelias
Retinoic acid	Hydrocephalus, microcephaly, heart defects, malformations of cranium, ear, face, and ribs, limb deformities, stillbirth
Spermicides	Limb reduction
Sulfonamide	Hypoplasia of limb or limb part, foot defects, urethral obstructions
Tetracycline	Hypoplasia of limb or limb part, clubfoot
Thalidomide	Heart defects, spine malformation, limb reduction (amelia, phocomelia), limb hypoplasia, duodenal stenosis or atresia, pyloric stenosis, microtia
Thioguanine	Missing digits
Tobacco	Growth retardation
Tolbutamide	Finger/toe syndactyly, absent toes, accessory thumb
Trifluoperazine	Transposition of great arteries, phocomelia
Trimethadione	Microcephaly, atrial septal defect, ventricular septal defect, low-set ears, broad nasal bridge, malformed hands, clubfoot, esophageal atresia, growth deficiency
Valproic acid	Lumbosacral meningomyelocele, microcephaly, wide fontanelle, tetralogy of Fallot, depressed nasal bridge, hypoplastic nose, low-set ears, small mandibles, oral cleft, growth deficiency

[a] Modified table reprinted from ref. 4 with permission.

TABLE 1.8. *Highly selected examples of sporadic and hereditary syndromes (5–7)*

Syndrome	Characteristics
Amniotic band	Early rupture of the amnion results in some combination of extremity amputation, edema, postural defects, body wall defects, facial clefts, scoliosis, neural tube defects, etc.
Limb-body wall complex	Failure of separation of the peritoneal cavity and chorionic cavity results in lack of free umbilical cord formation and persistence of abdominal contents in the chorionic cavity (extraembryonic coelom). Associated findings include scoliosis, limb defects, large body wall defects, neural tube defects, etc.
Beckwith-Wiedemann	This sporadically occurring syndrome results in macrosomia, macroglossia, large kidneys, omphalocele, and many other abnormalities.
Ivemark's	This sporadically occurring syndrome results in either polysplenia or asplenia (bilateral left or right sidedness) and in some combination of cardiac abnormalities, abnormal lung lobulation, and malpositioned stomach, liver, aorta, and inferior vena cava.
VATERS (VACTERL)	This sporadically occurring syndrome results in some combination of **V**ertebral anomalies, **V**entricular septal (and other cardiac) defects, **A**nal atresia, **T**racheo **E**sophageal fistula, **R**adial dysplasia, **R**enal abnormalities, and **S**ingle umbilical artery.
Meckel-Gruber	This autosomal recessive syndrome results in some combination of an encephalocele, polycystic kidneys, and polydactyly together with many other possible anomalies.
Achondroplasia	This autosomal dominant syndrome, which often occurs by mutation, includes a heterozygous variety with moderate limb shortening, mild macrocephaly, low nasal bridge, lumbar lordosis, etc., and a lethal homozygous variety with marked limb shortening, more severe macrocephaly, and a narrow thorax.
Caudal regression	This syndrome, which may occur with uncontrolled maternal diabetes mellitus, results from incomplete development of the caudal portion of the embryo and may include agenesis of the distal spine, distal bowel, and genitourinary structures and fusion or reduction abnormalities of the lower extremities.

References

1. Heinonen OP, Slone D, Shapiro S. *Birth defects and drugs in pregnancy*. Littleton, MA: Publishing Sciences Group, 1977.
2. Beer AE, Rayburn WF. Diagnosis and management of the malformed fetus, an invitational symposium: introduction to the symposium. *J Reprod Med* 1982; 27:549.
3. Hook EB. Rates of chromosome abnormalities at different maternal ages. *Obstet Gynecol* 1981;58:282.
4. Koren G, Edwards MB, Miskin M. Antenatal sonography of fetal malformations associated with drugs and chemicals: a guide. *Am J Obstet Gynecol* 1987;156:79.
5. Smith DW, Jones KL. *Recognizable patterns of human malformation*. Philadelphia: WB Saunders, 1982.
6. Romero R, Pilu G, Jeanty P, Ghidini A, Hobbins JC. *Prenatal diagnosis of congenital anomalies*. Norwalk, CT: Appleton & Lange, 1988.
7. Nyberg DA, Mahony BS, Pretorius DH. *Diagnostic ultrasound of fetal anomalies: text and atlas*. Chicago: Year Book Medical Publishers, 1990.

Chapter 2

ANOMALIES DETECTABLE BY ULTRASOUND OF THE FETUS

Although congenital anomalies are present in 6.5% of children, only a portion of those anomalies are detectable prenatally by obstetric ultrasound. A study of general obstetric ultrasound in the early and middle 1980s determined the varieties of anomalies that are commonly detectable. Those anomalies are present in only 0.7% to 0.8% of fetuses at a rate of 1.15 detectable anomalies per 100 fetuses (1). All commonly detectable anomalies from that study are major anomalies. Minor anomalies are virtually never detectable.

In the 1990s the varieties of commonly detectable anomalies should be more numerous than they were in the early 1980s. Since that time, equipment and experience have evolved considerably, and a standard fetal anatomy survey has been formally recommended. With these changes, if just clubfoot, facial clefts, and some cardiac malformations are added to the commonly detectable group, the percentage of fetuses with commonly detectable anomalies will increase to 1.5% to 1.7% at a rate of 2.3 anomalies per 100 fetuses (Table 2.1) (1,2). These figures do not include arrhythmias, choroid plexus cysts, or mild renal pyelectasis.

Even with this improvement, only one-fourth of the 6.5% of children with congenital anomalies would have anomalies commonly detectable by obstetric ultrasound. This rate of potential detection is not surprising when the nature of the anomalies not commonly detected is considered.

Included in the group not commonly detected are all minor anomalies, many of which, such as hernias, hypospadias, cleft gum, and extra ribs, are intuitively unlikely to be detectable by obstetric ultrasound. Also included are major anomalies that are difficult to resolve or define, such as cataracts and hip dislocation, and major anomalies that are always or often expressed too late for prenatal detection, such as pyloric stenosis and childhood tumors (see Table 2.1).

Some anomalies in the group with late expression, such as microcephaly or porencephaly, are easily detectable by obstetric ultrasound but at lower rates than reported postnatally. Presumably this discrepancy occurs be-

TABLE 2.1. *Detectability of fetal major anomalies (1978 to 1987)[a]*

Commonly detected	Increasingly detected	Uncommonly detected
Hydrocephalus	Cardiac	Syndactyly
Hydrops	Clubfoot	Hypoplastic muscle
Cystic hygroma-lymphedema	Facial cleft	Pyloric stenosis
Multicystic kidney		Dislocated hip
Meningomyelocele		Microcephaly
Anencephaly		Miscellaneous CNS
Hydronephrosis		Genital
Body wall defect		Cataract

[a] Selected congenital anomalies according to prenatal detectability by general obstetric ultrasound from 1978 to 1987 (1). Some uncommonly detected anomalies are not expressed until late in gestation or after birth. Others are difficult to detect or not sought on ordinary screening examinations.

cause in many cases the abnormalities appear too late for detection. Hence, although these anomalies are detectable when present prenatally, they are not considered commonly detectable according to known rates of postnatal occurrence.

The percentage of fetuses considered to have anomalies commonly detectable by ultrasound does not indicate the rate of detection that is actually achieved. That rate is determined by the portion of detectable anomalies actually detected, the additional detection of any usually undetectable anomalies, and the selection of the patient population. In the past, these factors have varied considerably from one laboratory to the next, particularly between referral and general ultrasound laboratories (1).

In the United States, ultrasound is usually performed only in selected patients according to indications rather than routinely in all patients. Hence, the prevalence of detectable anomalies may be increased in the resulting selected populations. On the other hand, this system may result in the performance of ultrasound at suboptimal times for the detection of some anomalies.

Because of this selection process, reported rates of detection of anomalies by obstetric ultrasound vary considerably according to the subpopulation of patients studied. The rates vary from 0.33% for a relatively low-risk group at about 16 weeks gestational age to 17% for a high-risk group with more advanced gestational ages (3,4).

As this is written, a large prospective study is being conducted in the United States to determine the rate of detection of fetal anomalies in obstetric patients who have no indications for ultrasound.

References

1. Hegge FN, Franklin RW, Watson PT, Calhoun BC. Fetal malformations commonly detectable on obstetric ultrasound. *J Reprod Med* 1990;35:391.
2. Benacerraf BR, Pober BR, Sanders SP. Accuracy of fetal echocardiography. *Radiology* 1987;165:847.
3. Hegge FN, Prescott GH, Watson PT. Sonography at the time of genetic amniocentesis to screen for fetal malformations. *Obstet Gynecol* 1988;71:522.
4. Campbell S. Ultrasound in obstetrics and gynecology: recent advances. *Clin Obstet Gynecol* 1983;10:475.

Chapter 3

IMPACT OF THE SONOGRAPHIC DIAGNOSIS OF FETAL ANOMALIES

Numerous diagnostic and therapeutic options are available following the sonographic diagnosis of fetal anomalies. Chromosomal analysis may be performed, either by amniocentesis or by percutaneous umbilical blood sampling, and may further define the abnormalities. Special monitoring of pregnancies may be arranged as appropriate. Special circumstances of delivery may be set up, such as early delivery, cesarean section, or the immediate availability of various specialists at the time of delivery. In other cases that appear to be hopeless, these measures may be avoided when premature labor or fetal distress occurs.

Active treatment of the fetus during pregnancy may occasionally be performed, such as fetal transfusion for hydrops or, rarely, experimental fetal surgery for diaphragmatic hernia or urinary tract obstruction. Nevertheless, termination of the pregnancy remains an important option during pregnancy in many cases. This option depends on the timing of discovery of the anomalies because it is quite limited after 22 to 24 weeks gestational age.

Unfortunately, in the United States, fetal anomalies often go undiscovered until the option of termination of the pregnancy has become limited. This is the case at least in part because ultrasound is ordinarily not per-

TABLE 3.1. *Time of discovery of anomalous fetuses when obstetric ultrasound is not ordered until specific indications arise*[a]

Gestational age at discovery		If late discovery, onset of indications that led to scan		If late discovery, onset of any indications	
≤22 weeks	≥23 weeks	≤22 weeks	≥23 weeks	≤22 weeks	≥23 weeks
33%	67%	28%	72%	43%	57%

[a] Modified table reprinted from ref. 2 with permission of The American College of Obstetricians and Gynecologists.

TABLE 3.2. *Outcome of pregnancies with fetal anomalies according to time of discovery[a]*

Outcomes	Discovery ≤22 weeks	Discovery ≥23 weeks
Termination	71%	14%
Survival	10%	50%
Cesarean section	6%	48%

[a] Modified table reprinted from ref. 2 with permission from The American College of Obstetricians and Gynecologists.

formed until specific indications occur, and those indications most commonly do not occur until relatively late during gestation (1,2).

According to a study of fetal anomalies discovered by obstetric ultrasound, only 33% are discovered before 23 weeks, usually because ultrasound is not performed earlier (Table 3.1). Furthermore, for those discovered after 23 weeks, the indications that lead to discovery are also present only after 23 weeks in 72%, and no indications are present until after 23 weeks in 57% (2).

In clinical practice this late discovery of fetal anomalies by the indication-based system of ordering obstetric ultrasound has a very important impact on the outcome of involved pregnancies. According to the study previously cited, patients with early discovery of fetal anomalies are much more likely to have their pregnancies terminated and much less likely to undergo cesarean section. Discovery of anomalies before 23 weeks is associated with termination in 71%, long-term survival in 10%, and cesarean section in 6%. Discovery after 23 weeks is associated with termination in 14%, long-term survival in 50%, and cesarean section in 48% (Table 3.2).

Programs such as maternal serum alpha-fetoprotein testing and genetic amniocentesis help to promote early discovery for some fetal anomalies but are not helpful for many others. Routine ultrasound at 18 to 20 weeks would address this issue for almost all anomalies, but its cost-effectiveness remains controversial. Large, well-designed studies that are now being conducted should help to resolve this issue.

References

1. *Consensus development conference: diagnostic ultrasound imaging in pregnancy.* Washington, DC: United States Department of Health and Human Services (NIH publication 84–667), 1984.
2. Hegge FN, Franklin RW, Watson PT, Calhoun BC. An evaluation of the time of discovery of fetal malformations by an indication-based system for ordering obstetric ultrasound. *Obstet Gynecol* 1989;74:21.

Chapter 4

RECOMMENDED FETAL ANATOMY SURVEY BY CLINICAL SOCIETIES

Radiologic, sonographic, and obstetric societies have all recommended that a systematic review of fetal anatomy be performed during second and third trimester obstetric ultrasound because of the potential to detect major fetal anomalies (1,2). These recommendations were issued in 1985 by the American College of Radiology (ACR), in 1986 by the American Institute of Ultrasound in Medicine (AIUM), and in 1988 by the American College of Obstetrics and Gynecology (ACOG). The ACR and AIUM recommendations were revised in 1990.

The 1985 ACR and 1986 AIUM guidelines, which are very similar, recommend that a study should include but not necessarily be limited to the cerebral ventricles, spine, stomach, urinary bladder, umbilical cord insertion site, and renal region (1). The 1988 ACOG guidelines also recommend examination of these structures but in addition recommend examination of the cranial configuration, cerebral midline, cerebellum, cardiac four chambers, and long bones of the extremities (2). The 1990 revised ACR and AIUM guidelines recommend the addition of the cardiac four chambers to their fetal anatomy survey (Table 4.1).

The inclusion of the additional items in the ACOG and revised ACR and AIUM guidelines appears to be appropriate when the prevalences of detectable anomalies and the experience with the fetal anatomy survey is considered (Tables 4.1, 4.2). In particular, the cardiac examination, which is included in the ACOG and revised ACR and AIUM guidelines, facilitates detection of some of the most common major fetal anomalies, although not all varieties are detectable by a four chamber view or even by a more complete examination.

All of the preceding guidelines recognize that it is unrealistic to expect complete accuracy in the detection of anomalies. On the other hand, cases that occur after these guidelines were issued will likely be judged in court by their standards. Furthermore, it is likely that if image documentation of a relevant area is not obtained, it will be assumed that the area was not examined (3).

TABLE 4.1. *Prevalences of selected commonly detectable fetal anomalies according to each step of the fetal anatomy survey as recommended by the AIUM or ACOG[a]*

Fetal structure visualized	AIUM 1986[b]	AIUM 1990[b]	ACOG 1988[b]	Prevalence of anomalies commonly detectable by ultrasound
Skull			X	1/750
Cerebral ventricles and midline	X	X	X	1/542[c]
Cerebellum			X	1/1,062
Orbits				1/1,712
Nose and lip				1/520
Spine	X	X	X	1/558
Heart (and thorax)		X	X	1/120[c]
Gastric fluid (and abdomen)	X	X	X	1/1,176
Renal region	X	X	X	1/384[c]
Cord insertion site	X	X	X	1/3,003
Urinary bladder	X	X	X	1/3,344
Extremities			X	1/457

[a] Prevalences are approximate because multiple references are used, midpoints of ranges are used, and anomalies expressed at multiple sites are variably listed singly or multiply according to complexity (4–8).
[b] Publication of recommendations.
[c] Choroid plexus cysts, cardiomegaly, arrhythmias, and mild renal pyelectasis are excluded from this determination.

TABLE 4.2. *Number of fetal structural abnormalities observed by each step of the fetal anatomy survey[a]*

Fetal anatomy survey step	Number of abnormalities
Skull	94
Cerebral ventricles and midline	166[b]
Cerebellum	35
Orbits	21
Nose and lip	47
Spine	159
Heart (and thorax)	211[b]
Stomach (and abdomen)	144
Kidneys	176[b]
Umblical cord insertion	70
Urinary bladder	28
Extremities	76
Step not recorded (edema and lymphedema)	98
All steps	1,325

[a] Emanuel Hospital, through 1990.
[b] Choroid plexus cysts, arrhythmias, secondary cardiomegaly, and mild pyelectasis are excluded from this determination.

These guidelines also recognize that when abnormalities are suspected, a specialized examination may be required (1). This examination, which may be called a referral or a directed, targeted, or level II examination, will presumably be done on high-risk patients at a site with demonstrated special competence to a level of complexity that exceeds the standard guidelines. The existence of this more complex type of examination does not indicate that nonreferral, nondirected, nontargeted, or level I examinations do not need to meet the guidelines. Indeed, the guidelines are specifically intended for these basic examinations.

References

1. Leopold GR. Editorial: antepartum obstetrical ultrasound guidelines. *J Ultrasound Med* 1986;5:241.
2. Technical Bulletin. American College of Obstetrics and Gynecology, No. 116. 1988.
3. Sanders R. Understanding the medical/legal risks in obstetrical ultrasound. *ACR Bull* 1986;42:6.
4. Heinonen OP, Slone D, Shapiro S. *Birth defects and drugs in pregnancy*. Littleton, MA: Publishing Sciences Group, 1977.
5. Romero R, Pilu G, Jeanty P, Ghidini A, Hobbins JC. *Prenatal diagnosis of congenital anomalies*. Norwalk, Ct: Appleton & Lange, 1988.
6. Nyberg DA, Mahony BS, Pretorius DH. *Diagnostic ultrasound of fetal anomalies: text and atlas*. Chicago: Year Book Medical Publishers, 1990.
7. Smith DW, Jones KL. *Recognizable patterns of human malformation*. Philadelphia: WB Saunders Company, 1982.
8. Hegge FN, Franklin RW, Watson PT, Calhoun, BC. Fetal malformations commonly detectable on obstetric ultrasound. *J Reprod Med* 1990;35:391.

Chapter 5

THE FETAL ANATOMY SURVEY

The fetal anatomy survey at Emanuel Hospital includes visualization of the skull, cerebral ventricles and midline, cerebellum, orbits, nose and upper lip, spine, cardiac four chambers, cardiac outflow tracts (optional), gastric fluid, kidneys, cord insertion site, urinary bladder, and extremities (Table 5.1). With the exception of the orbits, nose, and upper lip, all of these structures are included in the fetal anatomy survey recommended by the American College of Obstetrics and Gynecology's technical bulletin of 1988 (1).

This review of fetal anatomy is performed by the sonographer as a part of any basic ultrasound examination in the second or third trimester. In some high-risk pregnancies, a similar but more intense examination may be performed by the sonologist as well.

To obtain optimal results from the fetal anatomy survey, a sonographer needs to have an awareness of what fetal abnormalities may be found. The achievement of this awareness may seem to be an impossible task when the numerous varieties of anomalies and syndromes are considered. However, this task is greatly simplified by remembering small groups of specific structural abnormalities according to the portions of the fetal anatomy survey that are likely to detect them.

With this approach each step of the fetal anatomy survey becomes an active search for a small group of specific anomalies. As an examiner's experience increases, the number of anomalies specifically sought in each group gradually increases, and the entire process requires less conscious effort. In the following discussion of the technique of the anatomy survey, a somewhat arbitrary list of anomalies to be sought at each step by beginners is indicated in italics, and additional rarer, more complex, or secondary anomalies that may be sought are indicated as well (Table 5.1).

Skull

The entire cranium and overlying scalp are examined by a continuous sweep of the real-time image from the superior portion to the base. Photographic documentation is not obtained at this time because it is included

TABLE 5.1. *Fetal anomalies according to steps of the fetal anatomy survey*

Fetal anatomy survey	Anomalies particularly sought	Additional anomalies
Skull	Anencephaly/ exencephaly Encephalocele Lemon sign (spina bifida)	Reduced mineralization (with skeletal dysplasia) Scalp edema Abnormal contour (cloverleaf, etc.)
Cerebral ventricles and midline	Hydrocephalus Holoprosencephaly Hydranencephaly Abnormal cyst (see text) Abnormal hyperechoic region (see text)	Agenesis of corpus callosum
Cerebellum	Banana sign (spina bifida) Large cisterna magna (trisomy 18) Dandy-Walker malformation	
Orbits	Anophthalmia/ cyclopia Hypo- or hypertelorism Proptosis	
Nose and lip	Facial cleft Proboscis Absent or flat nose	Micrognathia Facial mass (teratoma, etc.)
Spine	Cystic hygroma Posterior nuchal thickening Kyphoscoliosis Spina bifida	Other neck mass (teratoma, etc.) Incomplete mineralization (with skeletal dysplasia) Sacral agenesis Sacral teratoma

Cardiac four chambers (and thorax)	Dextroposition (situs abnormality, diaphragmatic hernia)
	Cardiomegaly
	Septal defects
	Ventricular disproportion
	Valvular abnormality
		Arrhythmia
		Rhabdomyoma
		Pericardial effusion
		Extracardiac thoracic findings
		  Pleural effusion
		  Solid or cystic lung masses
		  Deformed ribs (lethal dwarf)
		  Subcutaneous edema

TABLE 5.1. *Continued*

Fetal anatomy survey	Anomalies particularly sought	Additional anomalies
Cardiac outflow tracts		Overriding aorta Truncus arteriosus Complete transposition Double outlet right ventricle Valvular stenosis or atresia Aortic coarctation or hypoplasia
Gastric fluid (and abdominal region)	Esophageal atresia Duodenal atresia Small bowel atresia Ascites Meconium peritonitis	Solid or cystic masses Subcutaneous edema Situs abnormality Calcifications
Kidneys	Hydronephrosis Multicystic Polycystic Dysplastic Agenesis	Hydroureter (with hydronephrosis) Duplication (with hydronephrosis) Urinoma (with obstruction) Isolated cysts Ectopia (pelvic kidney)
Cord insertion site	Gastroschisis Omphalocele Limb-body wall complex	Umbilical cord mass Single umbilical artery
Urinary bladder	Outlet obstruction No filling (renal anuria) Exstrophy or cloaca	
Extremities	Dwarfism (lethal, nonlethal) Reduction (amputation, various aplasia) Clubfoot	Polydactyly Syndactyly Clinodactyly Fractures Abnormal muscle Subcutaneous edema

in photographs of the biparietal diameter, cerebellum, and cerebral ventricles and midline.

Abnormalities particularly sought are *anencephaly or exencephaly* (absent cranium and absent or markedly abnormal cerebral hemispheres), *encephalocele* (cranial defect with herniated contents), and the *lemon sign* (bifrontal indentations suggesting spinal meningomyelocele). An awareness is also maintained, particularly in specific contexts, for other abnormalities such as deformed contour (cloverleaf skull, etc.), incomplete mineralization

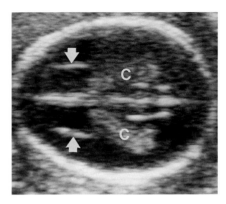

FIG. 5.1. Skull, lateral ventricles, and midline. A transverse image of the head at 18 weeks shows the skull, midline, anterior horns of the lateral ventricles (*arrows*), and choroid plexus (C) in the bodies and atria of the lateral ventricles.

(various skeletal dysplasias), and scalp edema (with hydrops or cystic hygroma-lymphedema).

Cerebral Ventricles and Midline

These structures are examined by a continuous sweep of the real-time image from the level of the anterior horns and bodies of the lateral ventricles to the level of the atria. A photograph is obtained of an image at the level of the anterior horns and bodies (Fig. 5.1). At early gestational ages, increased prominence of the lateral ventricles is an expected normal finding as long as the atria are less than 1 cm in diameter and the bodies are filled transversely by the choroid plexus (2,3).

Abnormalities particularly sought are *hydrocephalus* (dilated ventricles), *holoprosencephaly* (absent midline structures, deformed and fused lateral ventricles, deformed cortex), *hydranencephaly* (absent ventricles and cortex), *abnormal cysts* (choroid plexus, porencephalic, arachnoid, cystic-appearing vein of Galen aneurysm), and *abnormal hyperechoic regions* (calcifications, hemorrhage, infarction, teratoma). Awareness is maintained for other abnormalities such as altered ventricular configuration with agenesis of the corpus callosum.

Cerebellum

The contents of the posterior fossa are examined by sweeping a real-time transverse image of the cerebellar hemispheres and cisterna magna within a plane that includes the thalamus. A representative image is photographed (Fig. 5.2). Ordinarily, the cerebellum has a contiguous bilobed appearance, and the cisterna magna has an anterior-posterior depth of less than 1 cm and does not separate the cerebellar hemispheres (4). In the early and middle second trimester, the overlying skin is up to 0.5 cm thick (5).

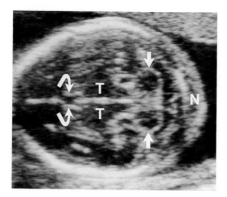

FIG. 5.2. Cerebellum. A transverse image of the head at 21 weeks shows the skull, cavum septi pellucidi (*curved arrows*), thalamus (T), cerebellum (*straight arrows*), and posterior nuchal region (N).

Abnormalities particularly sought are the *banana sign* (altered cerebellar configuration suggesting spinal meningomyelocele), a *large cisterna magna* (strongly associated with trisomy 18), and the *Dandy-Walker malformation* (posterior fossa cyst from an obstructed fourth ventricle separating the cerebellar hemispheres). An awareness is also maintained for abnormally thick posterior nuchal skin before about 20 weeks.

Orbits

The orbits are examined during a sweep of a coronal real-time image through the region of the face angled to include the orbits and forehead. In the third trimester, an anterior transverse image may be required because the increasingly mineralized bone becomes more difficult to penetrate. A representative image is photographed (Fig. 5.3). If an abnormality

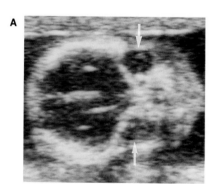
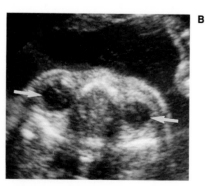

FIG. 5.3. Orbits. **A:** A coronal image of the face at 18 weeks shows the orbits (*arrows*) as well as portions of the facial bones and frontal skull. **B:** A transverse image of the face at 26 weeks shows the orbits (*arrows*).

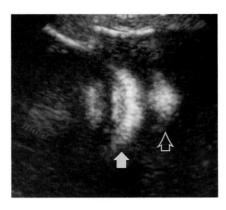

FIG. 5.4. Nose and upper lip. A coronal image of the face at 26 weeks shows the nose (*open arrow*), upper lip (*closed arrow*), and a portion of the lower lip.

is suspected, various measurements of the orbital regions may be compared to appropriate tables (6).

Abnormalities particularly sought are *anophthalmia* (absence of the orbits), *cyclopia* (single central orbit), *hypotelorism or hypertelorism* (abnormally spaced orbits), and *proptosis* (protruding orbital contents). Anophthalmia, hypotelorism, and cyclopia are particularly likely to be found when holoprosencephaly is present.

Nose and Lip

These structures are examined during a sweep of a real-time coronal image through the region of the face angled to include the nose, mouth, and chin. An image of the nose and upper lip is photographed (Fig. 5.4). If an abnormality of the chin is suspected, a sagittal image of the facial profile may be required as well.

Abnormalities particularly sought are a *proboscis* (fleshy protuberance instead of a nose), *abnormal nasal contour* (absent, flattened, single nostril), and *facial cleft* (median or lateral cleft lip, palate, or both). These abnormalities are particularly likely to be found when holoprosencephaly is present. Awareness is maintained for facial masses (teratoma, etc.). When chromosomal abnormalities are suspected, micrognathia (small chin) may be sought by additional views.

Spine

The spine is examined by sweeps of transverse and longitudinal (coronal or oblique sagittal) real-time images along its entire length. Particularly in the region of the sacrum, a diligent effort is made to include the overlying skinline on transverse and oblique sagittal images and to sweep through the skinline on coronal images. It may be necessary to push the fetus gently away from the uterine wall to accomplish this.

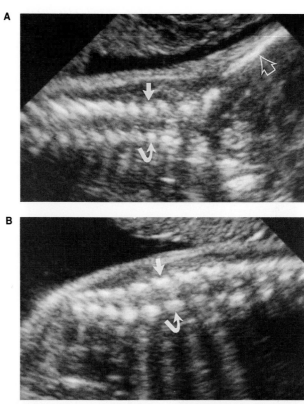

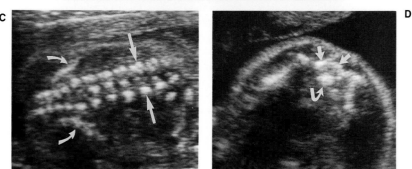

FIG. 5.5. Spine **A:** A sagittal image of the upper spine at 26 weeks shows the vertebral bodies (*curved arrow*), one row of posterior elements (*straight arrow*), the overlying skinline and part of the occipital skull (*open arrow*). **B:** A sagittal image of the lower spine at 26 weeks shows the vertebral bodies (*curved arrow*), one row of posterior elements (*straight arrow*), and the overlying skinline. **C:** A coronal image of the lower spine at 22 weeks shows the ilia (*curved arrows*) and the posterior elements (*straight arrows*) of the lumbar and sacral spine. **D:** A transverse image of the lower spine at 26 weeks shows the body (*curved arrow*) and two posterior elements (*straight arrows*) of a sacral vertebra, the ilia, and the overlying skinline.

A transverse image of the lower spine and longitudinal images of the upper and lower spine are photographed (Fig. 5.5). The transverse image includes the skinline, iliac wings, and posterior elements and body of the sacrum. The longitudinal images include the rows of right and left posterior elements if coronal or the skinline and rows of vertebrae and right or left posterior elements if sagittal.

For the cervical spine and adjacent regions, anomalies particularly sought are *posterior cystic hygroma* (large septated lymphatic fluid collection together with generalized subcutaneous lymphedema) and *posterior nuchal thickening* (thick skin that may be associated with Down syndrome). Awareness is maintained for other neck masses (teratoma, isolated cystic hygroma, etc.).

For the middle and lower spine and adjacent regions, anomalies particularly sought are *kyphoscoliosis* (abnormally curved spine such as with limb-body wall complex) and *spina bifida* (usually split lumbosacral posterior arches with exposed neural canal or cystic mass). Awareness is maintained for sacral teratoma (usually a large solid and/or cystic mass arising from the sacrum), sacral agenesis, and reduced mineralization (in the presence of skeletal dysplasia).

Cardiac Four Chambers

These structures are examined by sweeping an oblique transverse real-time image of the thorax through the cardiac chambers. If possible, the posterior portion of this real-time image is then swept cephalad from the atria to the left and then the right ventricular outflow tracts. Representative images of the cardiac four chambers and, if possible, the outflow tracts are photographed (Fig. 5.6). The cardiac rhythm is observed and may be recorded on an M-mode image. A more comprehensive cardiac examination is described in the chapter on normal expanded cardiac anatomic examination.

The appropriateness of cardiac position is determined by conscious comparison to the positions of the fetal spine and right and left sides. The cardiac size is assessed by comparison to the overall thoracic size. The right and left ventricles, atria, and atrioventricular valves are evaluated for symmetry. The interventricular and interatrial septa are examined for position and defects (remember that the interatrial septum contains the foramen ovale and is bowed to the left). If the outflow tracts are visualized, they are evaluated for a normal crossing position and similar size.

Anomalies particularly sought are *left diaphragmatic hernia* (heart displaced to the right by abdominal contents herniated into the left chest), *heart failure* (diffuse enlargement with myopathy, tachycardia, Rh incompatibility, etc.), *septal defects* (ventricular septal defect, atrioventricular canal, single ventricle), *ventricular disproportion* (hypoplastic left or right

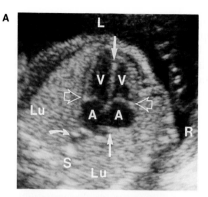

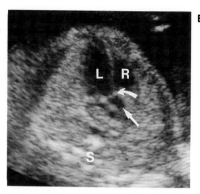

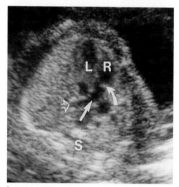

FIG. 5.6. Cardiac four chambers (and thorax). **A:** An oblique transverse image of the thorax at 21 weeks shows the atria (A), ventricles (V), interatrial and interventricular septa (*straight arrows*), and atrioventricular valves (*open arrows*) as well as the aorta (*curved arrow*), lungs (Lu), spine (S), and ribs (L, left; R, right). **B:** An oblique transverse image of the same fetus with slightly increased cephalad angulation of the posterior portion shows the ventricles (L, R), aortic valve (*curved arrow*), and aorta (*straight arrow*), which is crossing the pulmonary outflow region. **C:** An oblique transverse image of the same fetus with additional cephalad angulation of the posterior portion shows the ventricles (L, R), pulmonic valve (*curved arrow*), and pulmonary artery (*straight arrow*), which is crossing the aortic outflow region (left pulmonary artery, *Open arrow*).

ventricle, usually with valvular abnormalities), and *atrioventricular valvular abnormalities* (stenosis, atresia).

Mere evaluation for crossing and symmetry of the outflow tracts allows several outflow abnormalities to be sought as well, including *overriding aorta* (with tetralogy of Fallot), *truncus arteriosus* (single outflow tract), *complete transposition* (parallel rather than crossed outflow tracts), *double outlet right ventricle* (both outflow tracts from the right ventricle), *outflow valvular abnormalities* (stenosis, atresia), and *outflow asymmetry* (aortic coarctation, hypoplasia).

Awareness is also maintained for arrhythmias (particularly sustained tachycardia or bradycardia), focal myocardial abnormalities (calcifications, rhabdomyomas), and pericardial effusions. In addition awareness is maintained for noncardiac abnormalities, such as pleural effusions, solid or

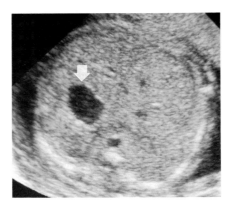

FIG. 5.7. Gastric fluid (and abdomen). A transverse image of the abdomen at 26 weeks shows left-sided gastric fluid (*arrow*) as well as other abdominal and skeletal structures and skin.

cystic lung masses (pulmonary sequestration or cystic adenomatoid malformation), constriction or deformity of the rib cage (particularly with lethal dwarfism or limb-body wall complex), or overlying subcutaneous edema (with hydrops or cystic hygroma-lymphedema).

Gastric Fluid

The region of the stomach and adjacent structures is examined by a continuous sweep of the real-time image through the abdomen. A representative image that includes gastric fluid is photographed (Fig. 5.7).

Anomalies particularly sought are *esophageal atresia* (absent gastric fluid), *duodenal atresia* (communicating fluid spaces in the stomach and dilated duodenum—"double bubble"), *small bowel atresia* (multiple tubular fluid spaces representing dilated loops of small bowel), *meconium peritonitis* (generalized or loculated fluid and calcifications from perforated bowel), and *ascites* (free fluid). Awareness is maintained for solid or cystic masses (ovarian cyst, etc.), calcifications, situs abnormalities, and overlying subcutaneous edema (with hydrops or cystic hygroma-lymphedema).

Kidneys

The entire renal regions are examined by a real-time sweep of a transverse image of the posterior abdomen. A representative image including both kidneys at the level of the renal pelves is photographed (Fig. 5.8). Occasionally, longitudinal images of the kidneys in the parasagittal or coronal planes are obtained as well. At gestational ages too early for renal visualization, a labeled photograph of the renal regions is obtained because abnormal fluid collections or cysts may still be detectable.

Anomalies particularly sought are *hydronephrosis* (dilated renal collecting system), *multicystic kidney* (nonfunctional kidney with extensive visualized

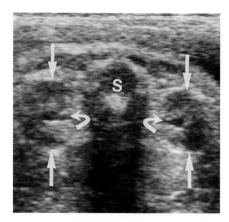

FIG. 5.8. Kidneys. A transverse image of the posterior abdomen at 37 weeks shows the right and left renal parenchyma (*straight arrows*) and renal pelves (*curved arrows*) as well as adjacent abdominal contents, the spine (S), and skin.

parenchymal cysts), *infantile polycystic kidneys* (enlarged, hyperechoic kidneys because of extensive parenchymal cysts too small to visualize), *dysplastic kidney* (dysfunctional kidney with abnormal parenchymal echogenicity), and *renal agenesis* (absent kidney). All of these anomalies may be bilateral, in which case oligohydramnios may be present as well.

Awareness is also maintained for ectopic kidney (pelvic kidney), hydroureter (dilated ureter), renal duplication (when hydronephrosis is present), urinoma formation (when obstruction is present), and isolated renal cysts.

Cord Insertion Site

This region is examined by a sweep of a real-time transverse image of the abdomen through the site of insertion of the umbilical cord into the anterior body wall. In addition the real-time image is swept throughout the adjacent amniotic fluid and/or flexed limbs to search for externalized abdominal structures, such as free-floating loops of bowel. A representative photograph of the umbilical cord entering the abdominal wall is obtained (Fig. 5.9). If the gestation is sufficiently advanced, an image of the three vessels of the umbilical cord may be photographed as well.

Anomalies particularly sought are *gastroschisis* (herniation of bowel through a paraumbilical body wall defect), *omphalocele* (herniation of abdominal structures, especially bowel and/or liver, into the base of the umbilical cord), and *limb-body wall complex* (umbilical cord confined by membranes, large body wall defect, extensive evisceration of abdominal contents, scoliosis, and limb abnormalities). Awareness is also maintained for abnormalities of the umbilical cord, such as solid or cystic masses or single umbilical artery.

A 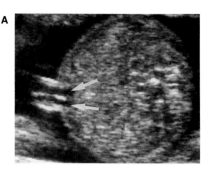 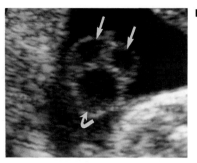 B

FIG. 5.9. Umbilical cord insertion site. **A:** A transverse image of the abdomen at 18 weeks shows the umbilical cord insertion site (*arrows*) as well as adjacent amniotic fluid, which is free of bowel. **B:** A transverse image of the umbilical cord at 35 weeks shows a single larger umbilical vein (*curved arrow*) and two smaller umbilical arteries (*straight arrows*).

Urinary Bladder

This structure is examined by a sweep of a real-time transverse image through the pelvis. A representative image is photographed (Fig. 5.10). Occasionally, follow-up images after allowing for filling of the bladder may be necessary.

Anomalies particularly sought are *outlet obstruction* (markedly enlarged bladder and/or thickened bladder wall together with bilateral hydrone-phrosis or renal dysplasia), *renal anuria* (nonvisualized bladder and oligo-hydramnios secondary to bilateral renal abnormalities, such as agenesis or multicystic dysplasia), and *bladder or cloacal exstrophy* (nonvisualized blad-der fluid and external pelvic mass representing an inverted bladder).

Extremities

Appropriate real-time images are used to determine the presence, shape, and relative size of the long bones of the upper and lower extremities and

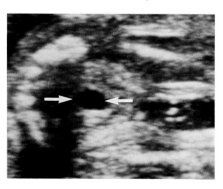

FIG. 5.10. Urinary bladder. A transverse image of the pelvis at 18 weeks shows fluid within the urinary bladder (*arrows*) as well as adjacent pelvic contents, pel-vic bones, and skin.

A 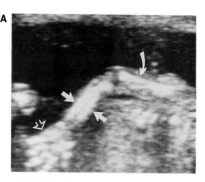 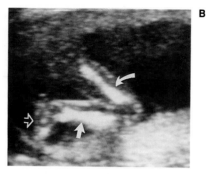 B

FIG. 5.11. Upper and lower extremities. **A:** An image of the upper extremity at 16 weeks shows the humerus (*curved arrow*), ulna and radius (*straight arrows*), and hand (*open arrow*). **B:** An image of the lower extremity at 16 weeks shows the femur (*curved arrow*), tibia (*straight arrow*), and foot (*open arrow*).

the presence of the hands and feet. At the present time, representative images are not ordinarily photographed because of the impracticality of obtaining comprehensive documentation in a few photographs. Perhaps a policy of obtaining limited documentation will be instituted in the future (Fig. 5.11).

Anomalies particularly sought include *dwarfism* (generalized shortening of long bones, particularly in lethal varieties), *reduction* (absence or hypoplasia of a limb or limb segment, such as distal amputation from amniotic bands, or developmental absence of internal segments ranging from isolated hypoplasia of a long bone to absence of all long bones), and *clubfoot*.

In appropriate clinical settings, awareness is also maintained for other anomalies such as polydactyly (extra digits), syndactyly (fused digits), clinodactyly (crossed digits), contractures, fractures (with osteogenesis imperfecta), abnormal appearance of muscle, and subcutaneous edema (with hydrops or cystic hygroma-lymphedema).

References

1. Technical bulletin. American College of Obstetrics and Gynecology, No. 116. May 1988.
2. Heiserman J, Filly RA, Goldstein RB. Effect of measurement errors on sonographic evaluation of ventriculomegaly. *J Ultrasound Med* 1991;10:121.
3. Benacerraf BR, Birnholz JC. The diagnosis of fetal hydrocephalus prior to 22 weeks. *J Clin Ultrasound* 1987;15:531.
4. Nyberg DA, Mahony BS, Hegge FN, et al. Enlarged cisterna magna and the Danby-Walker malformation: Factors associated with chromosome abnormalities. *Obstet Gyencol* 1991;77:436.
5. Benacerraf BR, Barss VA, Laboda LA. A sonographic sign for the detection in the second trimester of the fetus with Down's syndrome. *Am J Obstet Gynecol* 1985;151:1078.
6. Jeanty P, Cantraine F, Cousaert E, et al. The binocular distance: A new way to estimate fetal age. *J Ultrasound Med* 1984;3:241.

Chapter 6

OTHER FETAL ANATOMY

Many structures not specifically sought by the fetal anatomy survey are nevertheless identifiable by obstetric ultrasound. Sometimes recognition of these normal structures is important to avoid confusion about findings on the fetal anatomy survey. In a normal fetus, for example, the lateral margin of the cerebral cortex may be mistaken for the lateral margin of an enlarged lateral ventricle and lead to a mistaken diagnosis of hydrocephalus. Or, in an abnormal fetus with renal agenesis, the normal adrenal glands may be mistaken for the kidneys and lead to a failure to diagnose the abnormality correctly.

Abnormalities of these structures are occasionally identified on the fetal anatomy survey because they are strikingly visible (ovarian cysts, etc.) or because of displacement of adjacent structures (pulmonary cystic adenomatoid malformation, etc.). Also, when selected anomalies are found among the structures of the basic fetal anatomy survey, some additional structures may be sought as part of an extended survey. For example, with some cardiac abnormalities, it may be important to define the position and status of the liver, spleen, abdominal aorta, and inferior vena cava.

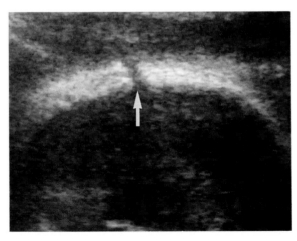

FIG. 6.1. Cranial suture. An image of a portion of the cranium at 27 weeks shows a cranial suture (*arrow*).

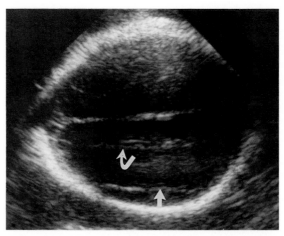

FIG. 6.2. Lateral margin of the cerebral cortex. A transverse image of the head at 26 weeks shows the lateral margin of the cerebral cortex (*straight arrow*) as well as structures near the lateral margin of the cerebral ventricle (*curved arrow*).

Selected fetal structures not specifically sought by the fetal anatomy survey but identifiable by ultrasound include the cranial sutures (Fig. 6.1), lateral margin of the cerebral cortex (Fig. 6.2), choroid plexus (Fig. 6.3), lens of the eye (Fig. 6.4), ear (Fig. 6.5), scalp hair (Fig. 6.6), chin (Fig. 6.7), tongue (Fig. 6.8), hypopharynx (Fig. 6.9), trachea (Fig. 6.10), lungs (Fig. 6.11), liver (Fig. 6.12), gall bladder (Fig. 6.13), adrenal gland (Fig. 6.14), bowel (Fig. 6.15), spinal cord (Fig. 6.16), genitals (Fig. 6.17), and digits of the hands and feet (Fig. 6.18).

A 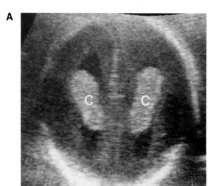 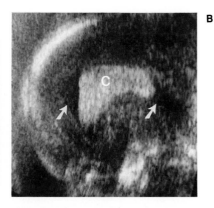 B

FIG. 6.3. Choroid plexus. **A:** A transverse image of the head at 19 weeks shows the choroid plexus (C) as well as fluid within the lateral ventricles. **B:** A parasagittal image of the head at 19 weeks shows the choroid plexus (C) and fluid within the lateral ventricle (*arrows*).

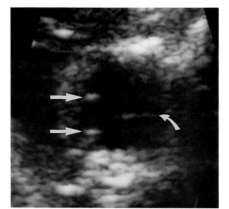

FIG. 6.4. Lens of the eye. A transverse image of the eye at 24 weeks shows the lateral and medial margins of the lens (*straight arrows*) along with the hyaloid artery (*curved arrow*), which will regress *in utero*.

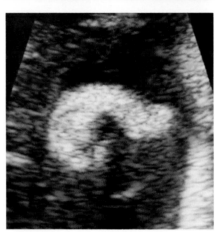

FIG. 6.5. Ear. A parasagittal image at 33 weeks shows the ear.

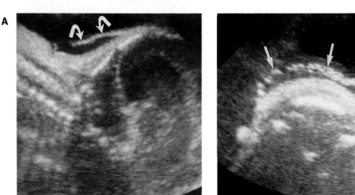

FIG. 6.6. Scalp hair. **A:** A posterior sagittal image of the head and neck in the third trimester shows an echogenic line at the free margin of scalp hair (*arrows*). **B:** A posterior transverse image of the inferior head shows an irregular echogenic line at the free margin of scalp hair (*arrows*).

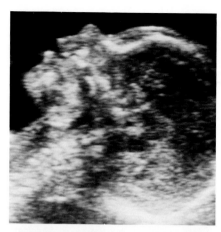

FIG. 6.7. Chin. An anterior sagittal image of the facial profile at 22 weeks shows the chin, lips, nose, and forehead.

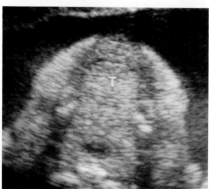

FIG. 6.8. Tongue. An anterior transverse image of the face at 26 weeks shows the tongue (T).

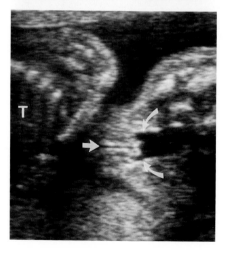

FIG. 6.9. Hypopharynx. A coronal image of the neck at 23 weeks shows fluid within the hypopharynx and piriform sinuses (*curved arrows*) and extending to the trachea (*straight arrow*). T, thorax.

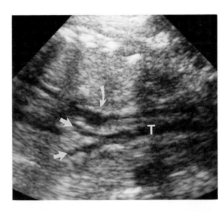

FIG. 6.10. Trachea. A coronal image of the thorax at 21 weeks shows the trachea (T), right and left bronchi (*straight arrows*), and a portion of the aortic arch (*curved arrow*).

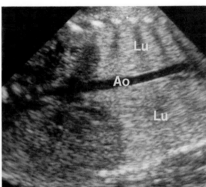

FIG. 6.11. Lungs. A coronal image of the thorax at 26 weeks shows the lungs (Lu) and aorta (Ao).

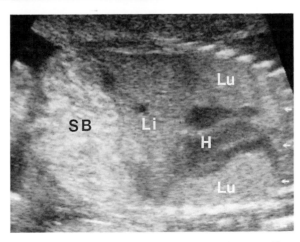

FIG. 6.12. Liver. A coronal image of the abdomen and thorax at 18 weeks shows the liver (Li) as well as the lungs (Lu), heart (H), and small bowel (SB).

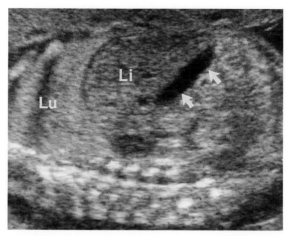

FIG. 6.13. Gall bladder. A parasagittal image of the abdomen and thorax at 22 weeks shows the gall bladder (*arrows*) and the lung (Lu), liver (Li), and small bowel.

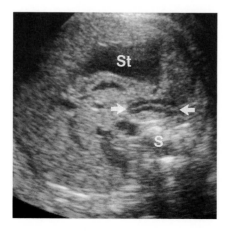

FIG. 6.14. Adrenal gland. A transverse image of the abdomen in the third trimester shows the adrenal gland (*arrows*). St, stomach; S, spine.

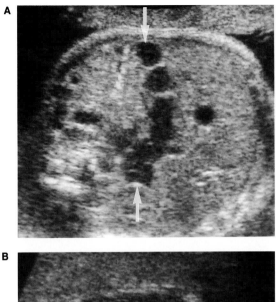

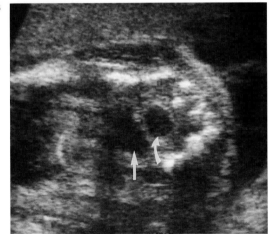

FIG. 6.15. Bowel. **A:** A transverse image of the abdomen at 34 weeks shows the transverse colon (*arrows*). **B:** A transverse image of the pelvis at 23 weeks shows a prominent rectosigmoid colon (*curved arrow*) adjacent to the sacrum that should not be mistaken for the urinary bladder (*straight arrow*).

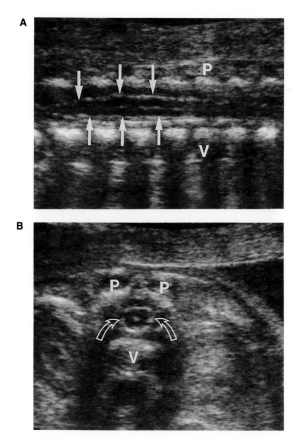

FIG. 6.16. Spinal cord. **A:** A posterior sagittal image of the spine at 25 weeks shows the distal spinal cord (*arrows*) as it tapers to form the conus medullaris between the vertebral bodies (V) and posterior spinal arches (P). **B:** A posterior transverse image of the spine at 25 weeks shows the spinal cord (*arrows*) between the vertebral body (V) and posterior spinal arch (P).

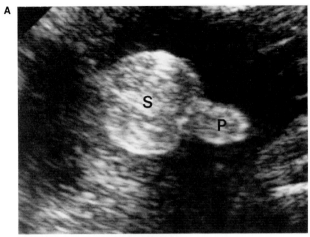

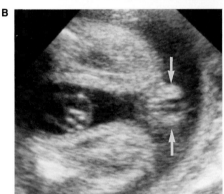

FIG. 6.17. Genitals. **A:** A transverse image at 35 weeks at the level of the genitals shows the scrotum (S) and penis (P) in a male. **B:** A transverse image at 28 weeks at the level of the genitals shows the labia majora (*arrows*) in a female.

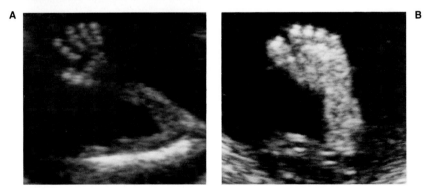

FIG. 6.18. Digits of the hands and feet. **A:** An image at 16 weeks shows the digits of the hand. **B:** An image at 20 weeks shows the digits of the foot.

Chapter 7

SCANNING TECHNIQUE

The fetal anatomy survey is a real-time examination. The interpreter may confirm that a real-time survey performed by a sonographer is adequate by reviewing photographed images. If the survey is abnormal, however, the interpreter should confirm and characterize the abnormality by direct real-time imaging.

The general principles important in any kind of ultrasound examination are equally important for the fetal anatomy survey. Images should be properly zoomed so that the region of interest fills the image rather than a small portion at the top or elsewhere within the image (Fig. 7.1). Gentle pressure on the transducer may be necessary to improve the image by compressing intervening soft tissue.

Image quality should be maximized by proper transducer selection. The appropriate balance must be determined between better resolution at higher frequencies and better penetration and lower noise at lower frequencies. A sector transducer may be used to improve access around intervening structures or to press through excess adipose tissue. A linear array transducer may be used to improve resolution or to provide a wider near field. A curved array transducer may serve as a compromise between these

A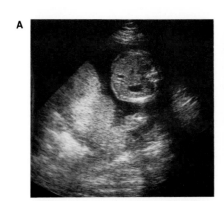 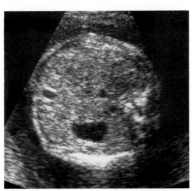B

FIG. 7.1. Zooming of images. **A:** An image of the fetal abdomen at 23 weeks is inadequately zoomed. **B:** A properly zoomed image of the same fetal abdomen optimally fills the space available for display.

41

two extremes. Sometimes more than one transducer is required during a single examination.

Images should ordinarily be obtained in a standard sequence according to a protocol. This process facilitates review by an interpreter and guards against inadvertent omissions, particularly if scanning is interrupted. Occasional exceptions to this approach may be made when the urinary bladder appears to be about to empty or when the heart, spine, or kidney appear to be transiently in an optimal position for imaging.

Certain pitfalls for beginners should be avoided. (1) Avoid making abnormal structures appear normal. For example, the four chamber image of a heart with a ventricular septal defect can be made to appear normal by including only an uninvolved portion of the septum (Fig. 7.2). (2) Avoid attributing an incomplete anatomy survey to adverse scanning circumstances. The inability to image a structure may be the first clue that it is abnormal. (3) Avoid including unrecognized ambiguous regions on images of the organs of interest. It is necessary to be aware of all portions of a photographed image, not just the target organ. Ambiguities should be resolved by real-time imaging and not photographed if insignificant.

An experienced examiner can usually complete the entire fetal anatomy survey for a basic obstetric sonogram in 5 to 10 minutes. However, in the presence of adverse scanning circumstances such as maternal obesity, oligohydraminos, late gestational age, multiple gestations, or persistent suboptimal fetal position, the examination may be prolonged, and special techniques may be required.

For an obese patient, it may be necessary to use a lower frequency transducer and to change the log compression curves. A sector transducer usually provides a better image with less noise than other transducers because

A
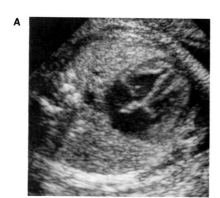
B
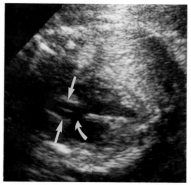

FIG. 7.2 Making the abnormal appear normal. **A:** A cardiac four chamber image at 21 weeks appears to be normal. **B:** A slightly modified image in the same patient shows a ventricular septal defect (*curved arrow*) and an overriding aorta (*straight arrows*).

its small footprint permits better compression of adipose tissue. Also, images are considerably improved by scanning through the thinner regions of the maternal body wall, particularly the paraumbilical region, the suprapubic region below the panniculus, and to a lesser extent the lateral regions. Until late in the gestation, most scanning can be done through these regions, particularly if the fetus and the body wall are gently moved as required.

Minor problems of fetal position can often be solved by gently moving the fetus or by changing from a linear array to a sector transducer. For example, gentle pressure may be sufficient to turn a fetal part that is too oblique for optimal imaging. However, more intense pressure and other difficult manipulations of the fetus are not justified for a basic ultrasound examination.

More elaborate procedures may be required when a fetus at risk for a particular anomaly remains in a persistent suboptimal position. If the inaccessible fetal part is positioned deeply and posteriorly within the maternal pelvis, it may be necessary to lower the head of the scanning table and to have the patient roll onto her side in order to allow gravity to move the fetal part.

Having the patient roll from side to side may also improve access to the ventral or dorsal side of the fetus for scanning of the heart or spine. Increasing or decreasing distention of the maternal urinary bladder may occasionally improve access to fetal structures. Sometimes nonstandard images alone, such as multiple oblique images, will be adequate to replace an inaccessible standard image (Fig. 7.3). It may occasionally (though rarely) be necessary to schedule the patient for a repeat examination.

A 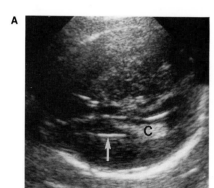 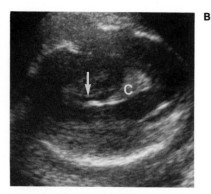 B

FIG. 7.3. Nonstandard images because of adverse fetal position. **A:** An oblique image of the head at 24 weeks shows the left lateral ventricular margin (*arrow*) and choroid plexus (C). **B:** A more sharply oblique image of the same head shows the right ventricular margin (*arrow*) and choroid plexus (C). Rarely, these images may be used in place of the standard transverse image for a fetal head deep in the pelvis.

For marked polyhydramnios scanning may be improved by changing the maternal position so the fetus rolls closer to the transducer. For oligohydramnios, multiple gestations, and late gestational age, special techniques may have limited usefulness, and the last resort may be increased persistence on the part of the examiner.

While performing the fetal anatomy survey, a good sonographer strives to maintain a professional, friendly interaction with the patient. Special care should be taken to avoid statements that needlessly add to a patient's anxiety. Even simple statements about fetal structure or expressions of uncertainty are easily misinterpreted by concerned patients.

When an anomaly is found, the fetal anatomy survey may be modified in several ways in order to characterize abnormal findings completely. Examination of the abnormal structure is often best deferred to the end of the fetal anatomy survey. This practice may help to avoid omissions in the remainder of the survey and may help defer questions to the end of the examination.

Ordinarily, images of the anomaly should be obtained in multiple planes to define it optimally and to determine its relationship to adjacent structures. In addition commonly associated patterns of abnormalities of other structures should be particularly sought. For this purpose the examination may be expanded to include structures not on the basic anatomy survey.

The anomaly is often best displayed on selected unzoomed images that include a large portion of the fetus or possibly the whole fetus for scale and orientation (Fig. 7.4). These images are particularly useful during review of the images by nonsonographers, such as clinicians or the patient. It may

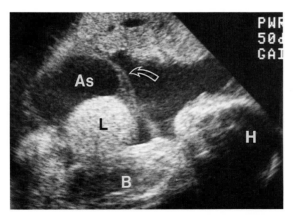

FIG. 7.4. Unzoomed image of a fetus with an anomaly. A relatively unzoomed anterior sagittal image of an omphalocele (*arrow*) at 28 weeks includes the fetal head and body to provide orientation and scale for nonsonographers who may review the image. H, head; B, body; L, liver; As, ascites.

be helpful to leave an appropriate image frozen on the monitor at the completion of the examination for this purpose.

If possible, abnormal findings are not discussed with the patient until the end of the examination. Discussion of abnormalities before they are completely defined may obviously cause incorrect or inappropriate statements to be made. In addition the distraction of an understandably intense discussion may undermine the examiner's performance of the remainder of the examination. In the worst case, the patient may be too upset to allow completion of the examination.

The abnormal findings should be communicated to the referring physician as soon as possible for determination of the course of action to be taken. This is particularly important in centers that have a team approach to anomalies that may involve referral to counselors, geneticists, perinatologists, and other specialists. The patient can ordinarily be presented with an appropriate management plan or actually initiate the plan before leaving the department.

If a possible anomaly is encountered that cannot be adequately characterized or managed locally, the patient should be promptly referred to a center that can do so. Delay of referral may limit management options such as termination or timely chromosomal analysis. Also, it may needlessly handicap the referral sonographer because examination of the fetus may become increasingly difficult near term.

Chapter 8

ONSET OF VISUALIZATION OF FETAL ANATOMY AND ANOMALIES

The fetal anatomy survey has been recommended for sonograms at 14 menstrual weeks or more (second or third trimester sonograms) (1,2). Because some anomalies may be identifiable, use of the fetal anatomy survey this early appears to be justifiable. With transabdominal ultrasound, however, many anomalies are likely to be missed because of the small size of some structures, the evolving appearance of other structures, and the incomplete expression of some anomalies.

By 16 weeks most structures of the fetal anatomy survey may be reasonably well visualized, although state-of-the-art equipment and special transducer selection may be required. Images of the nose and lip, heart, and kidneys may be poorly defined, however, particularly if scanning circumstances are adverse. These structures will ordinarily become well visualized between 16 and 20 weeks (Table 8.1). At that point most anomalies are readily detectable, although a few, such as intestinal obstruction, hydrops, and hydranencephaly, may not be detectable because of late expression (3).

A review of our experience tends to confirm the usefulness of the fetal anatomy survey early in the second trimester for the detection of at least some anomalies. For many kinds of anomalies, earliest detection was at 13 to 15 weeks, and for most remaining kinds earliest detection was at 16 to 17 weeks (Table 8.2). However, anomalies involving dilated bowel were not detected before 24 weeks.

The time of detection for most kinds of anomalies appears to be related more to the time ultrasound is ordered than to the time of earliest detectability. In our series neural tube defects and body wall defects tended have early detection times because maternal serum alpha-fetoprotein screening led to early ultrasound. Most other kinds of anomalies had intermediate detection times. However, several kinds of anomalies tended to have late detection times because of late expression or occurrence in organs hard to define at early gestational ages (Table 8.3).

TABLE 8.1. *Onset of visualization of fetal structures according to gestational age*

≤16 Weeks	16–20 Weeks	≥24 Weeks
Skull	Nose, lips	Dilated bowel
Ventricles	Heart	
Cerebellum	Kidneys	
Orbits		
Spine		
Stomach		
Cord insertion		
Urinary bladder		
Extremities		

TABLE 8.2. *Earliest gestational age at discovery for selected fetal anomalies at Emanuel Hospital (1978–1987)*

13–15 Weeks	16–17 Weeks	22+ Weeks
Cystic hygroma-lymphedema	Hydrocephalus	Gastrointestinal
Anencephaly	Other brain	Miscellaneous
Encephalocele	Skull	
Spine	Face	
Body wall	Meningomyelocele	
Renal	Cardiac structure	
Urinary bladder	Diaphragmatic hernia	
Extremities		
Hydrops		

TABLE 8.3. *Fetal anomalies according to likelihood of early detection (before 22 weeks) (Emanuel Hospital, 1978–1987)[a]*

40–86% Early detection	21–39% Early detection	0–20% Early detection
Cystic hygroma-lymphedema	Hydrocephalus	Other brain
Anencephaly	Diaphragmatic hernia	Face, skull
Encephalocele	Hydronephrosis	Cardiac structure
Meningomyelocele	Other renal	Bowel obstruction
Other spine	Urinary bladder	Hydrops
Body wall	Extremities	Miscellaneous
	Tumor	

[a] Early detection occurred in only 33% of all anomalies overall because early sonograms were not obtained unless indications were present. Most anomalies with high early detection rates were found because of maternal serum alpha-fetoprotein screening. Most anomalies with low early detection rates had late clinical expression or findings difficult to resolve on early ultrasound.

References

1. Leopold GR. Editorial: antepartum obstetrical ultrasound guidelines. *J Ultrasound Med* 1986;5:241.
2. Technical bulletin. American College of Obstetrics and Gynecology, No. 116. 1988.
3. Hegge FN, Franklin RW, Watson PT, Calhoun BC. An evaluation of the time of discovery of fetal malformations by an indication-based system for ordering obstetric ultrasound. *Obstet Gynecol* 1989;74:21.

Atlas: Sonographically Identifiable Fetal Anomalies at Each Step of the Fetal Anatomy Survey

Chapter 9

THE SKULL

Anencephaly

A

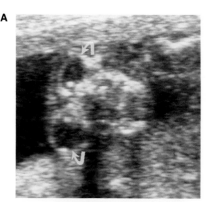

B

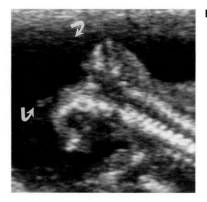

C

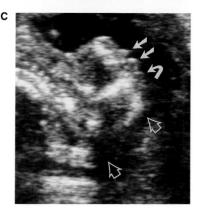

FIG. 9.1. Anencephaly. **A:** A coronal image of the facial bones and orbits (*arrows*) at 19 weeks shows complete absence of the cranium and cerebral hemispheres above the level of the orbits. **B:** A coronal image of the cervical spine in the same fetus shows complete absence of the cranium and cerebral hemispheres (*arrows*) above the level of the base of the skull. **C:** A sagittal image of the neck and head of another fetus at 19 weeks shows complete absence of the cranium above the level of the base of the skull (*open arrows*). *Straight arrows,* lips; *curved arrows,* nose.

The cranium and cerebral ventricles are absent. Some amorphous brain tissue may be present at the base of the skull. This is a lethal anomaly.

Anencephaly (*contd.*)

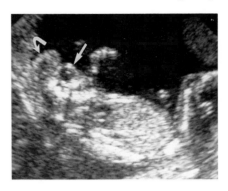

FIG. 9.2. Anencephaly with some brain tissue. A sagittal image of the fetus at 17 weeks shows amorphous brain tissue (*curved arrow*) at the base of the skull but complete absence of the cranium and complete absence of recognizable cerebral hemispheres above the level of the orbit (*straight arrow*).

Exencephaly (Acrania)

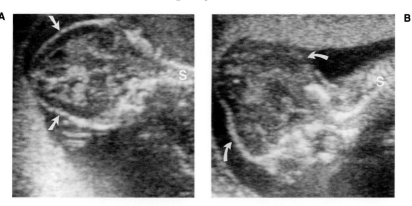

FIG. 9.3. Exencephaly (acrania). **A:** A coronal image of the head and cervical spine (S) at 18 weeks shows the presence of an abnormal brain with hyperechoic margins (*arrows*) but complete absence of the cranium. **B:** A sagittal image of the head and cervical spine (S) in the same fetus shows the presence of an abnormal brain with hyperechoic margins (*arrows*) but complete absence of the cranium.

The cranium is absent, but the brain, which is abnormal, is present. This is a lethal anomaly.

Encephalocele

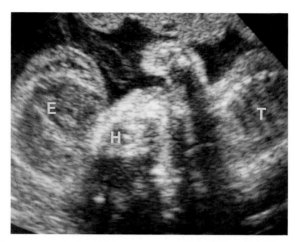

FIG. 9.4. Large encephalocele. A coronal image of the fetus at 26 weeks shows a large, mostly solid encephalocele (E) and associated microcephaly (H). T, thorax.

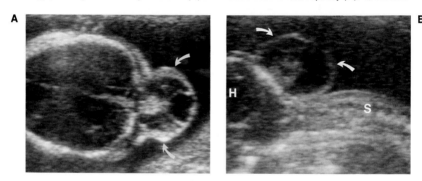

FIG. 9.5. Posterior encephalocele. **A:** A transverse image of the head at 21 weeks shows a mixed solid and cystic posterior encephalocele (*arrows*). **B:** A posterior sagittal image of the head (H) and upper thorax of the same fetus shows a mixed solid and cystic posterior encephalocele (*arrows*). S, spine.

Brain tissue is herniated through a cranial defect. This anomaly is likely to result in death or severe impairment.

Encephalocele (*contd.*)

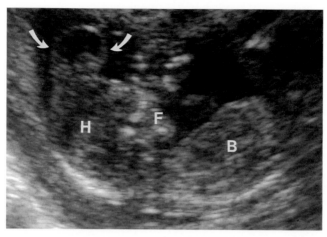

FIG. 9.6. Anterior encephalocele. An anterior sagittal image of the fetus at 15 weeks shows a mixed solid and cystic anterior encephalocele (*arrows*). H, head; F, face; B, body.

Lemon Sign

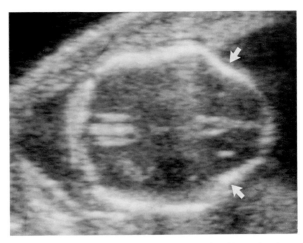

FIG. 9.7. Lemon sign. A transverse image of the head at 18 weeks shows bifrontal indentations (*arrows*) that cause the cranium to have a configuration suggestive of a lemon, a finding that was associated with the presence of a meningomye-locele.

Bifrontal indentations of the skull result in a configuration on a transverse image similar to that of a lemon. This finding strongly suggests the presence of a spinal meningomyelocele.

Incomplete Mineralization

A

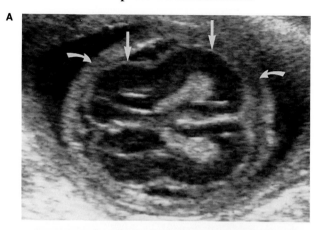

B

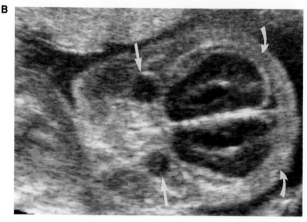

FIG. 9.8. Incomplete mineralization. **A:** A transverse image of the head at 19 weeks shows a lack of the usual hyperechoic appearance of the cranium (*curved arrows*) that results in better than usual visualization of the cerebral hemispheres (*straight arrows*) in a fetus with osteogenesis imperfecta type II. **B:** A coronal image of the head in the same fetus shows a lack of the usual hyperechoic appearance of the cranium (*curved arrows*), orbits (*straight arrows*), and facial bones.

Incomplete mineralization results in reduced or absent ultrasound visualization of the cranium. This finding may occur with some forms of lethal dwarfism (osteogenesis imperfecta type II, achondrogenesis, and hypophosphatasia).

Scalp Edema

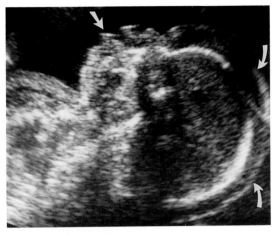

FIG. 9.9. Scalp edema with hydrops. An anterior sagittal image of the head at 24 weeks shows thickened subcutaneous tissue of the scalp (*curved arrows*) and face (*straight arrow*) in a fetus with immune hydrops.

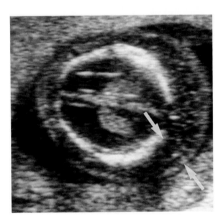

FIG. 9.10. Scalp edema with cystic hygroma. A transverse image of the head at 16 weeks shows markedly thickened subcutaneous tissue of the scalp (*arrows*) in a fetus with a posterior cystic hygroma and generalized lymphedema shown on other images.

The scalp is abnormally thickened because of edema from hydrops with congestive heart failure or because of generalized lymphedema with a posterior cystic hygroma.

Cloverleaf Skull

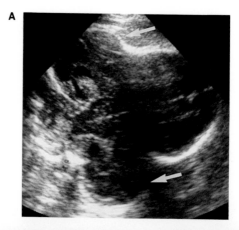

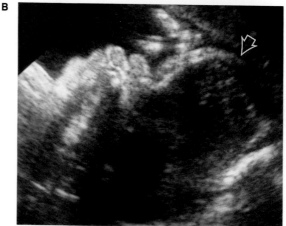

FIG. 9.11. Cloverleaf skull. **A:** A coronal image of the head at 31 weeks shows marked bitemporal prominences (*arrows*). **B:** An anterior sagittal image of the head of the same fetus shows marked prominence of the forehead (*arrow*) as well as an abnormal appearance of the lips and nose.

This deformity includes a tower forehead, marked bitemporal prominences, and distorted facial features. It is probably related to premature closure of multiple sutures. This anomaly may occur with lethal (thanatophoric) dwarfism or with other skeletal abnormalities.

Other Abnormal Skull Contours

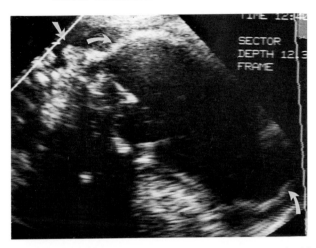

FIG. 9.12. Elongated skull from extreme molding. An anterior sagittal image of the head at 26 weeks shows marked elongation of the cranium (*curved arrows*) in a fetus held in a fixed position for several weeks by a rigid uterus with multiple fibroids. Postnatal follow-up revealed no evidence of cranial synostosis. *Straight arrow*, nose.

The skull may be deformed because of other patterns of premature closure of sutures or because of mechanical constriction, such as constriction by amniotic bands.

Microcephaly

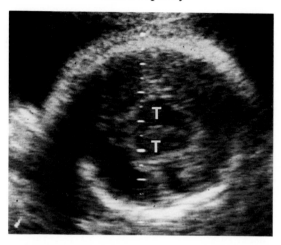

FIG. 9.13. Microcephaly. A transverse image of the head at 29 weeks shows a biparietal diameter of only 5.9 cm (7.3 cm expected) as well as fused thalami (T) with holoprosencephaly in a fetus with trisomy 13.

The head circumference is more than three standard deviations below the mean for true gestational age. This anomaly is identified by fetal biometry rather than the fetal anatomy survey, although it may be suspected during imaging. Associated intracranial anomalies, such as holoprosencephaly, may be apparent.

Macrocephaly

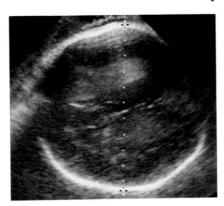

FIG. 9.14. Macrocephaly. A transverse image of the head at 34 weeks shows a biparietal diameter of 10.6 cm (8.5 cm expected) in a fetus with homozygous achondroplasia.

The head circumference is abnormally large for the true gestational age. This anomaly is identified by fetal biometry rather than the fetal anatomy survey, although it may be obvious during imaging. Associated intracranial anomalies, such as hydrocephaly or hydranencephaly, are likely to be apparent.

Chapter 10

THE CEREBRAL VENTRICLES AND MIDLINE

Normal Early Lateral Ventricular Prominence

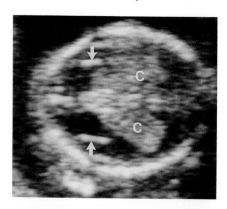

FIG. 10.1. Normal lateral ventricles at 15 weeks. A transverse image of the head shows normal relative prominence of the anterior horns (*arrows*) and bodies of the lateral ventricles and normal complete transverse filling of the bodies of the lateral ventricles by choroid plexus (C).

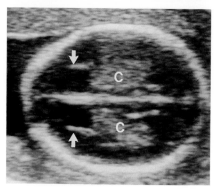

FIG. 10.2. Normal lateral ventricles at 18 weeks. A transverse image of the head shows somewhat decreased normal relative prominence of the lateral ventricles (*arrows*) since 15 weeks but continued complete transverse filling of the bodies of the lateral ventricles by choroid plexus (C).

Normal Early Lateral Ventricular Prominence (*contd.*)

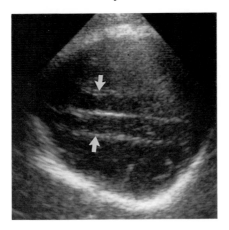

FIG. 10.3. Normal lateral ventricles at 30 weeks. A transverse image of the head shows the position of the lateral ventricles (*arrows*) and indicates that they are no longer relatively prominent compared to the cerebral cortex.

The lateral ventricles and choroid plexus are quite prominent relative to the cerebral cortex early in the second trimester. This relative prominence gradually diminishes because the width of the cerebral cortex increases but that of the lateral ventricles does not. Because the lateral ventricles do not change, complete transverse filling of their bodies by choroid plexus and widths of 1.0 cm or less for their atria are stable normal findings (1).

Hydrocephalus

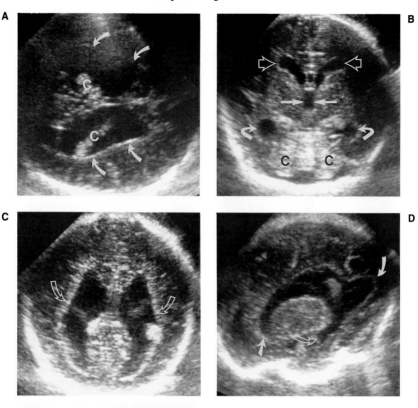

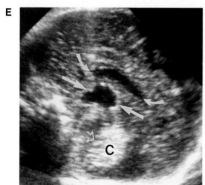

FIG. 10.4. Mild hydrocephalus. The configuration of the mildly dilated ventricular system is demonstrated in multiple images of the head of a 34-week fetus with trisomy 18. **A:** A transverse image shows the lateral ventricles (*arrows*) incompletely filled by choroid plexus (C). **B:** A coronal image shows the bodies (*open arrows*) and temporal horns (*curved arrows*) of the lateral ventricles, the third ventricle (*straight arrows*), and the cerebellum (C). **C:** A posterior coronal image shows the lateral ventricle atria (*arrows*), which contain small portions of choroid plexus. **D:** A parasagittal image shows the entire lateral ventricle, including the anterior horn (*straight arrow*), occipital horn (*closed curved arrow*), and temporal horn (*open curved arrow*). **E:** A midsagittal image shows the third ventricle (*straight arrows*) as well as the region of the nondilated fourth ventricle (*open arrow*), the cerebellum (C), and the cavum septi pellucidi and cavum vergae (*curved arrows*).

Hydrocephalus (*contd.*)

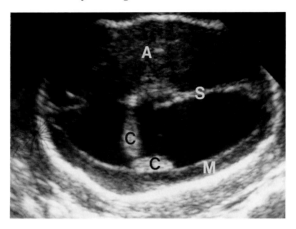

FIG. 10.5. Severe hydrocephalus. A transverse image of the head at 22 weeks shows severely dilated lateral ventricles, a thin mantle of cerebral cortex (M), and a diminished appearance of the choroid plexus (C). A, artifact; S, septum pellucidum.

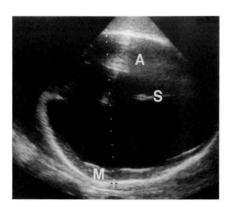

FIG. 10.6. Severe hydrocephalus causing macrocephaly. A transverse image of the head at 37 weeks shows severely dilated lateral ventricles, a thin mantle of cerebral cortex (M), and an incomplete septum pellucidum (S). A, artifact. The biparietal diameter is 11.7 cm.

The cerebral ventricles, particularly the lateral ventricles, are abnormally dilated. During early to middle gestation, this finding is differentiated from normal relative lateral ventricular prominence by lack of complete filling of the bodies by choroid plexus and by atrial diameters of greater than 1.0 cm. When discovered prenatally, this anomaly usually results in death or severe disability.

Hydrocephalus (*contd.*)

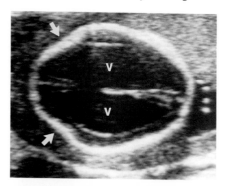

FIG. 10.7. Hydrocephalus with meningomyelocele. A transverse image of the head at 19 weeks shows dilated lateral ventricles (V) together with the bifrontal indentations (*arrows*) of the lemon sign.

A

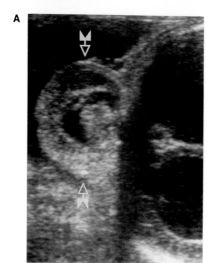

B

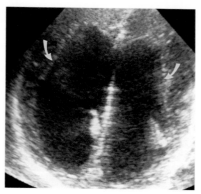

FIG. 10.8. Hydrocephalus with encephalocele. **A:** A posterior transverse image of the head at 34 weeks shows a mixed solid and cystic encephalocele (*arrows*). **B:** A posterior coronal image of the head of the same fetus shows dilated lateral ventricular atria (*arrows*) and a diminished appearance of the choroid plexus.

Hydranencephaly

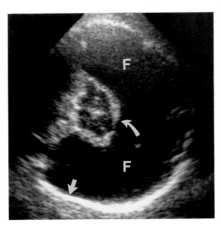

FIG. 10.9. Hydranencephaly. A lateral coronal image of the head at 37 weeks shows complete replacement of the cerebral hemispheres by fluid (F), resulting in absence of the cortical mantle (*straight arrow*) and minimal residual brain tissue at the base of the skull (*curved arrow*).

The cerebral hemispheres are absent, probably because of extensive infarction from a vascular incident that occurred after normal embryogenesis. This anomaly results in death or short-term survival with severe disability.

Holoprosencephaly

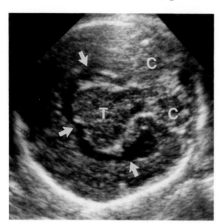

FIG. 10.10. Holoprosencephaly—complete cortical mantle. A transverse image of the head at 31 weeks shows an abnormal monoventricular lateral ventricular system (*arrows*) that communicates across the midline, surrounds prominent fused thalami (T), and is completely covered by cerebral cortex. C, cerebellum.

Division of the brain into cerebral hemispheres and lateral ventricles is incomplete. In alobar and semilobar varieties, the interhemispheric fissure is completely or partly absent, the lateral ventricles are completely or partly fused, the thalami are completely or partly fused, and accompanying abnormalities of the eyes, nose, and mouth are likely. This anomaly is likely to be associated with chromosomal abnormalities, and it results in death or, rarely, survival with severe disability.

Holoprosencephaly (*contd.*)

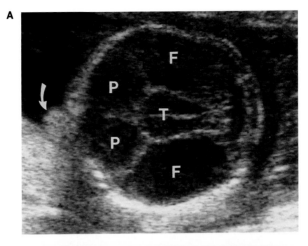

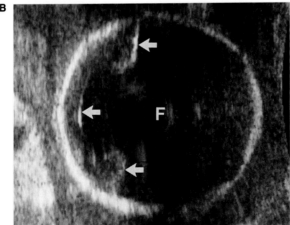

FIG. 10.11. Holoprosencephaly—incomplete cortical mantle. **A:** A transverse image of the head near the base of the skull at 22 weeks shows prominent fused thalami (T), only anterior cerebral parenchyma (P), fluid (F) within a monoventricular system filling the remainder of the cranium, and a proboscis (*arrow*). **B:** A somewhat higher transverse image of the head of the same fetus shows the edge of an incomplete mantle of cerebral cortex (*arrows*) that covers only the lower frontal part of the cranium. F, fluid.

Calcification

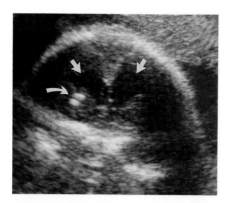

FIG. 10.12. Focal periventricular calcification. An anterior coronal image of the head at 28 weeks shows two focal periventricular calcifications (*curved arrow*) and mild dilatation of the anterior horns of the lateral ventricles (*straight arrows*) in association with cytomegalovirus infection.

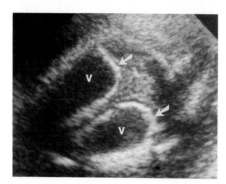

FIG. 10.13. Diffuse periventricular calcification. A posterior coronal image of the head at 25 weeks shows diffuse periventricular calcification (*arrows*) and dilated atria of the lateral ventricles (V) in association with cytomegalovirus infection.

Calcium is deposited in a diffuse or focal pattern, usually in the periventricular cerebral parenchyma in association with cytomegalovirus or toxoplasma infection.

Tumor

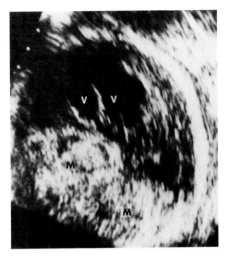

FIG. 10.14. Malignant tumor. A coronal image of the head at 37 weeks shows ventriculomegaly (V) and a large hyperechoic mass (M) found to be a teratoma. (From ref. 2, with permission.)

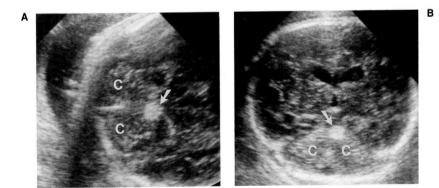

FIG. 10.15. Benign tumor. **A:** A transverse image of the head at 33 weeks shows a small hyperechoic focus (*arrow*) near the cerebellum (C) that was found to be a lipoma on postnatal imaging. **B:** A coronal image of the head of the same fetus shows mildly prominent lateral and third ventricles as well as the hyperechoic focus (*arrow*) and cerebellum (C).

A hyperechoic or complex mass is present within the brain.

Hemorrhage or Hemorrhagic Infarction

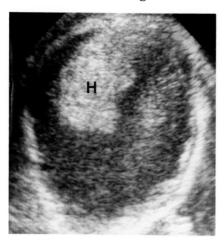

FIG. 10.16. Hemorrhagic infarction. A transverse image of the head at 24 weeks shows a large hyperechoic focal lesion (H) that appeared during follow-up of a fetus with nonimmune hydrops.

In the acute phase, hyperechoic focal lesions are present within the brain in either a vascular or a subependymal and interventricular distribution. The hyperechoic parenchymal lesions may be precursors to porencephalic cysts or hydranencephaly.

Porencephalic Cyst

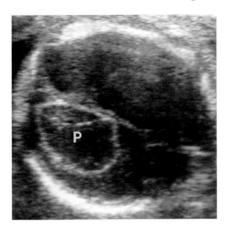

FIG. 10.17. Porencephalic cyst. A transverse image of the head of the fetus shown in Fig. 10.15 two weeks later shows transformation of the lesion from hyperechoic to cystic (P).

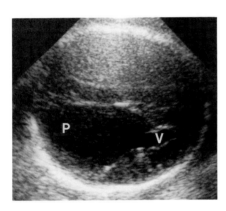

FIG. 10.18. Porencephalic cyst contiguous with the ventricle. A transverse image of the head at 33 weeks shows a large posterior cyst (P), which is contiguous with the anterior portion of the lateral ventricle (V).

A cyst that contains cerebrospinal fluid is present within the cerebral parenchyma. This cyst may communicate with the cerebral ventricles.

Arachnoid Cyst

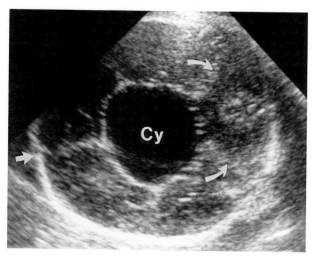

FIG. 10.19. Arachnoid cyst. A transverse image of the head at 36 weeks shows a large cyst (Cy) in the midline (*straight arrow*) anterior to the cerebellum (*curved arrows*).

An arachnoid-lined cyst that compresses adjacent structures is present within the intracranial region.

Choroid Plexus Cyst

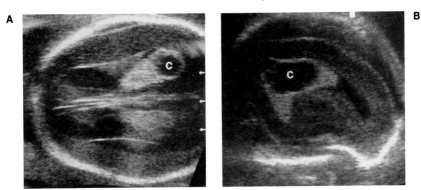

FIG. 10.20. Choroid plexus cyst. **A:** A transverse image of the head at 18 weeks shows a choroid plexus cyst (C). **B:** A sagittal image of the head at 19 weeks shows a large choroid plexus cyst (C).

One or more cysts are transiently present in the choroid plexus of the lateral ventricles during the second trimester. These cysts resolve spontaneously within several weeks and have no functional significance. Their presence, however, is associated with up to a 3% likelihood of trisomy 18. If the cysts are small and unilateral, and if an extensive anatomy survey is otherwise unremarkable, this likelihood of trisomy 18 appears to be substantially reduced.

Vein of Galen Aneurysm

A 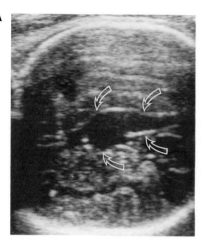 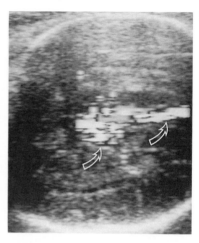 B

FIG. 10.21. Vein of Galen aneurysm. **A:** A transverse image of the head at 33 weeks shows an anechoic dilated vein of Galen (*arrows*). **B:** A similar image in the same patient with the addition of color Doppler (photographed with gray scale only) shows turbulent flow within the dilated vein of Galen (*arrows*).

As a result of an arteriovenous malformation, the vein of Galen is abnormally dilated. Characteristic abnormal blood flow is present within the venous aneurysm.

Agenesis of the Corpus Callosum

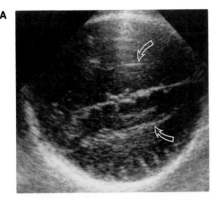

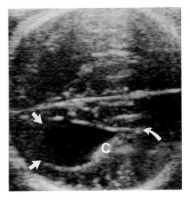

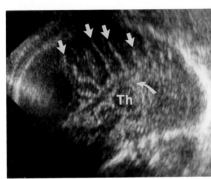

FIG. 10.22. Agenesis of the corpus callosum. **A:** A transverse image of the head at 32 weeks shows prominent separation of the anterior portions of the lateral ventricles (*arrows*). **B:** An oblique transverse image of the head of the same fetus shows beaklike narrowing of the anterior portion (*curved arrow*) and dilatation of the posterior portion (*straight arrows*) of the lateral ventricle. C, choroid plexus. **C:** A midsagittal image of the head of the same fetus shows sulci (*straight arrows*) radiating superiorly from the region of the third ventricle (Th) and no visualized corpus callosum (*curved arrow*) or cingulate sulcus.

The corpus callosum is completely or partly absent. Associated abnormalities include altered shape of the lateral ventricles, high position of the third ventricle (which may result in a prominent midline cyst), and sulci radiating superiorly from the third ventricle in place of the usual anteroposterior cingulate sulcus. The prognosis with this anomaly is quite variable.

References

1. Siedler DE, Filly RA. Relative growth of the higher brain structures. *J Ultrasound Med* 1987;6:573–6.
2. Lipman SP, Pretorius DH, Rumack CM, Manco-Johnson ML. Fetal intracranial teratoma: US diagnosis of three cases and a review of the literature. *Radiology* 1985;157:491–4.

Chapter 11

THE CEREBELLUM

Banana Sign

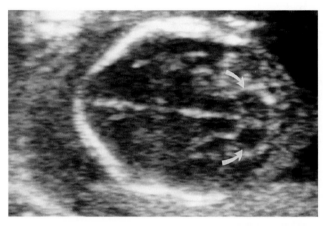

FIG. 11.1. Banana sign. A transverse image of the head at 19 weeks shows a curved rather than a bilobed cerebellum (*arrows*) with a convex posterior margin suggestive of a banana. This finding was associated with the presence of a meningomyelocele.

The posterior cerebellar margin is smoothly curved and convex, rather than bilobed. As a result, the cerebellar configuration on a transverse image is similar to that of a banana. This finding strongly suggests the presence of the Arnold-Chiari malformation secondary to a spinal meningomyelocele.

Large Cisterna Magna

A

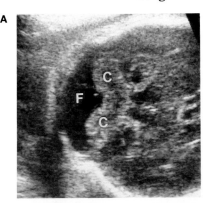

B

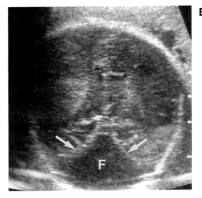

C

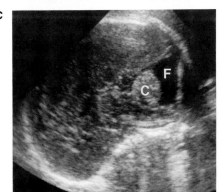

FIG. 11.2. Large cisterna magna. **A:** A transverse image of the head at 35 weeks shows an increased anteroposterior diameter of the fluid-filled cisterna magna (F) posterior to the cerebellum (C) in a fetus with trisomy 18. **B:** A coronal image of the head of the same fetus shows a prominent fluid-filled cisterna magna (F) below the tentorium (*arrows*). **C:** A sagittal image of the head of the same fetus shows a prominent fluid-filled cisterna magna (F) posterior to the cerebellum (C).

The anteroposterior diameter of the fluid-filled cisterna magna is abnormally increased. As a rule of thumb, a diameter of greater than 1 cm is considered abnormal, although the normal range depends somewhat on gestational age. This finding suggests cerebellar dysgenesis secondary to trisomy 18, particularly if other anomalies are identified (1).

Dandy-Walker Malformation

A 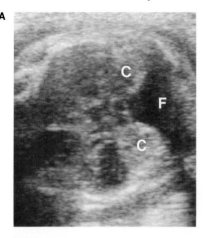 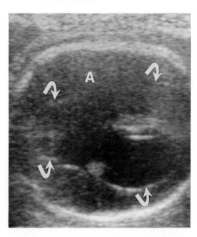 B

FIG. 11.3. Dandy-Walker malformation. **A:** A transverse image of the head at 29 weeks shows a posterior fossa cyst (F) between the widely separated cerebellar hemispheres (C). **B:** A transverse image of the head of the same fetus shows associated dilatation of the lateral ventricles (*arrows*). A, artifact.

A large posterior fossa cyst, which originates from an obstructed fourth ventricle, causes abnormal separation of the cerebellar hemispheres and partial or complete absence of the cerebellar vermis. The lateral ventricles, which are upstream from the fourth ventricle, are ordinarily dilated as well. This anomaly is likely to result in death or severe disability.

Reference

1. Nyberg DA, Mahony BS, Hegge FN, et al. Enlarged cisterna magna and the Dandy-Walker malformation: factors associated with chromosome abnormalities. *Obstet Gynecol* 1991;77:436–42.

Chapter 12

THE ORBITS

Anophthalmia

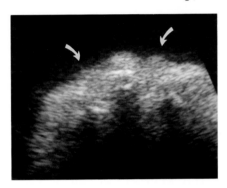

FIG. 12.1. Anophthalmia. An anterior transverse image of the head at 32 weeks shows no visualized orbits (*arrows*) at the expected level in a fetus with holoprosencephaly and trisomy 13.

The orbits are absent, possibly in association with holoprosencephaly. The clinical outcome is likely to be determined by associated findings, such as holoprosencephaly and chromosomal abnormalities.

Cyclopia

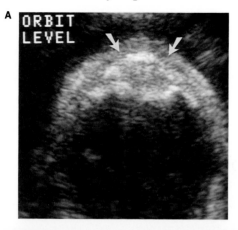

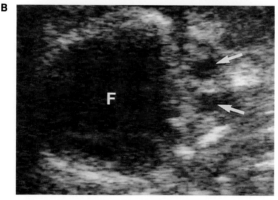

FIG. 12.2. Cyclopia. **A:** An anterior transverse image of the head at 24 weeks in a fetus with holoprosencephaly shows a single orbit (*arrows*) that contained no eyes on postmortem examination. **B:** An anterior coronal image of the head of a different fetus at 16 weeks shows extreme hypotelorism of abnormally small eyes (*arrows*) compatible with cyclopia in a fetus with trisomy 13 that also had holoprosencephaly and a proboscis. F, fluid.

In cyclopia the eyes are fused or closely adjacent to each other. An associated proboscis is likely to be present. These findings often occur in association with holoprosencephaly and chromosomal abnormalities.

Hypotelorism

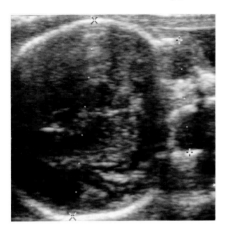

FIG. 12.3. Hypotelorism. A transverse image of the head at 28 weeks angled through the biparietal region and the orbits shows a small binocular distance (*graticules*) and interocular distance (not marked) compared to the biparietal distance (*graticules*) in a fetus with trisomy 18.

In hypotelorism the distance between the eyes is decreased. This anomaly often occurs in association with holoprosencephaly and chromosomal abnormalities.

Proptosis

A
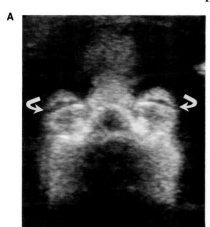

B
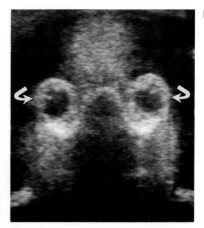

C
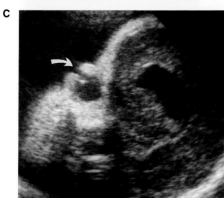

FIG. 12.4. Proptosis. **A, B:** Coronal images through the face at 26 weeks show prominence of the eyelids (*arrows*) and eyes (*arrows*) in a fetus with a cloverleaf skull. **C:** A parasagittal image of the head of the same fetus shows prominence of the eyes and eyelids (*arrow*). (From ref. 1, with permission.)

The eye protrudes abnormally from the orbit. This finding may occur with cloverleaf skull.

Reference

1. Mahony BS, Hegge FN. The face and neck. In: Nyberg DA, Mahony BS, Pretorius DH, eds. *Diagnostic ultrasound of fetal anomalies: text and atlas.* Chicago: Year Book Medical Publishers, 1990;203–61.

Chapter 13

THE NOSE AND LIPS

Arhinia

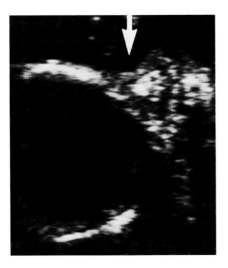

FIG. 13.1. Arhinia. An anterior sagittal image of the head at 25 weeks shows absence of the nose (*arrow*) in a fetus also found to have anophthalmia but no proboscis in association with holoprosencephaly.

The nose is absent. This finding may occur in association with orbital abnormalities and the presence of a proboscis together with holoprosencephaly and chromosomal abnormalities.

Proboscis

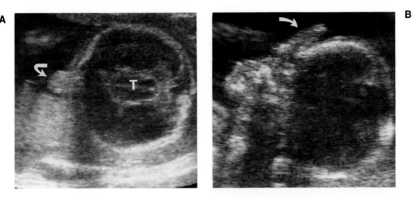

FIG. 13.2. Proboscis. **A:** A transverse image of the head at 22 weeks shows a proboscis (*arrow*) adjacent to the inferior frontal skull in a fetus also found to have monoventricular hydrocephalus, fused thalami (T), arhinia, and anophthalmia in association with holoprosencephaly. **B:** An anterior sagittal image of the head in the same fetus shows a proboscis (*arrow*) and arhinia.

A cylindrical appendage is present above or below the level of the orbits. This finding may occur in association with arhinia and cyclopia or other orbital abnormalities together with holoprosencephaly and chromosomal abnormalities.

Single Nostril

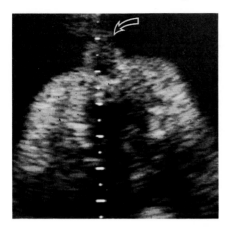

FIG. 13.3. Single nostril. An anterior transverse image of the head at 29 weeks shows a nose with only a single nostril (*arrow*) in a fetus with holoprosencephaly.

The nose contains only one nostril. This finding may occur in association with orbital abnormalities together with holoprosencephaly and chromosomal abnormalities.

Flattened Nose

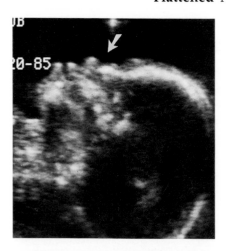

FIG. 13.4. Flattened nose. An anterior sagittal image of the head at 20 weeks shows a flattened nose (*arrow*) in association with maternal coumadin exposure. (From ref. 1, with permission.)

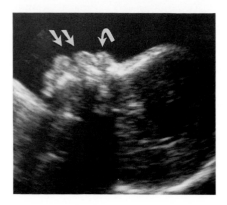

FIG. 13.5. Abnormal nose and lips with cloverleaf skull. An anterior sagittal image of the head at 26 weeks shows a nose (*curved arrow*) that appears small or flattened relative to the prominent lips (*straight arrows*) and forehead.

The nose is flattened with some syndromes. The nose may appear flattened relative to the prominent lips with cloverleaf skull.

Median Facial Cleft

A

B

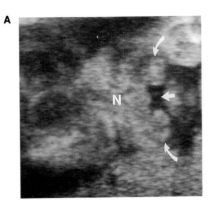
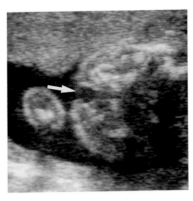

FIG. 13.6. Median facial cleft. **A:** A coronal image of the face at 23 weeks shows a quadrangular median defect (*straight arrow*) of the upper lip (*curved arrows*) that extends across the midline. N, region of nose. **B:** A transverse image of the face of the same fetus shows extension of the cleft into the palate (*arrow*).

A large cleft that extends through the midline is present within the medial upper lip and palate. This anomaly often occurs with holoprosencephaly and chromosomal abnormalities.

Lateral Facial Cleft

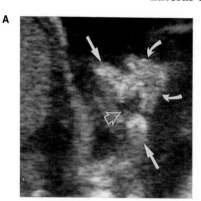
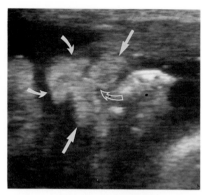

FIG. 13.7. Lateral facial cleft. **A:** A coronal image of the face at 26 weeks shows a lateral defect with a gap (*open arrow*) in the upper lip (*straight arrows*) below one nostril of the nose (*curved arrows*). **B:** A coronal image of the face of another fetus at 30 weeks shows a lateral defect without a gap (*open arrow*) in the upper lip (*straight arrows*) below one nostril of the nose (*curved arrows*).

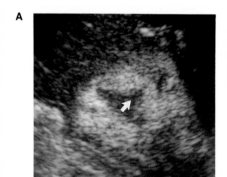
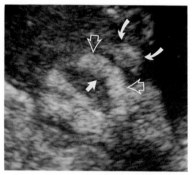

FIG. 13.8. Facial pseudocleft. **A:** A coronal image of the face at 35 weeks with the lips and nose pressed against the uterine wall shows the region of the frenulum (*arrow*) of the upper lip in a pattern falsely suggestive of a cleft. **B:** A repeat coronal image of the face of the same fetus with the nose and lips no longer pressed against the uterine wall shows no cleft (*straight arrow*) in the same region of the upper lip (*open arrows*). *Curved arrows,* nose.

A cleft is present within the lateral upper lip, the palate, or both.

Macroglossia

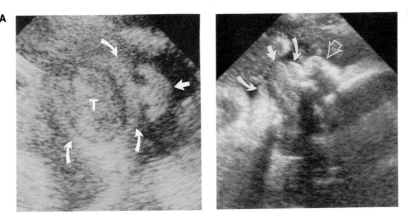

FIG. 13.9. Macroglossia. **A:** A coronal image of the face at 38 weeks shows an enlarged tongue (T) protruding through the lips (*curved arrows*) of a fetus with Beckwith-Wiedemann syndrome. *Straight arrow*, nose. **B:** A sagittal image of the face of the same fetus shows an enlarged tongue (*straight arrow*) protruding through the lips (*curved arrows*). *Open arrow*, nose.

An enlarged tongue that protrudes from the mouth is present, particularly in association with Beckwith-Wiedemann syndrome.

Micrognathia

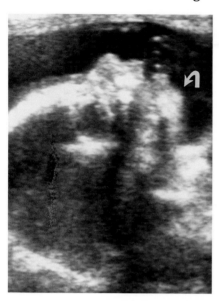

FIG. 13.10 Micrognathia. A sagittal image of the face at 26 weeks shows a somewhat rounded profile with a somewhat small chin (*arrow*) in a fetus with trisomy 18.

The lower jaw is abnormally small with some syndromes, such as trisomy 18.

Facial Mass

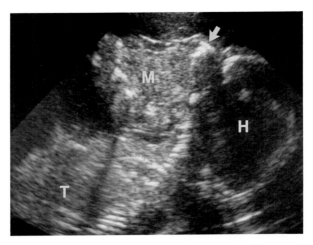

FIG. 13.11. Facial teratoma (epignathus). An anterior sagittal image of the head (H) and thorax (T) at 20 weeks shows a large mass (M) extending from the face just below the level of the maxilla (*arrow*). On postmortem examination, the mass originated in the pharynx and protruded through the mouth and nose.

Masses such as teratomas or isolated cystic hygromas may involve portions of the face. A mass that severely compromises the airway is likely to result in neonatal death.

Reference

1. Hegge FN, Prescott GH, Watson PT. Fetal facial abnormalities identified during obstetric sonography. *J Ultrasound Med* 1986;5:679–84.

Chapter 14

THE SPINE: UPPER PORTION

Normal Cervical Spine

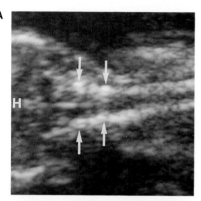

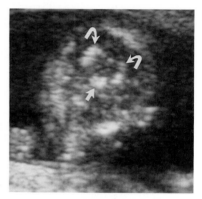

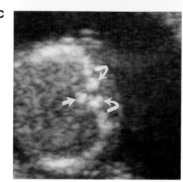

FIG. 14.1. Normal cervical spine. **A:** A coronal image of the cervical spine at 15 weeks shows normal spreading of the posterior elements (*arrows*) as they approach the head (H). **B:** A transverse image of an upper cervical vertebra of the same fetus shows the ossification centers of the body (*straight arrow*) and posterior elements (*curved arrows*). **C:** A transverse image of a thoracic vertebra of the same fetus with a similar scale shows the ossification centers of the body (*straight arrow*) and posterior elements (*curved arrows*).

The posterior elements of the cervical spine diverge as they approach the base of the skull. This is a normal finding that should not be confused with a neural tube defect.

Posterior Nuchal Thickening

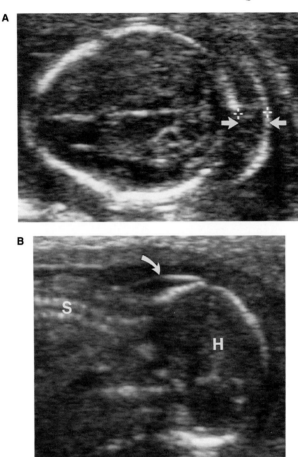

FIG. 14.2. Posterior nuchal thickening. **A:** A transverse image of the head angled through the cerebellum at 19 weeks shows abnormal thickening (0.8 cm) of the soft tissue overlying the skull (*arrows*) in a fetus with early hydrops. **B:** A posterior sagittal image at 15 weeks shows abnormal thickening of the soft tissue overlying the lower skull and upper neck (*arrow*) in a fetus with trisomy 21. H, head; S, spine.

The skin of the posterior neck is abnormally thickened (greater than 0.5 cm). In the mid trimester, this finding is strongly suggestive of trisomy 21 (1). Technical factors, normal variability, and early hydrops may also result in this finding.

Posterior Cystic Hygroma

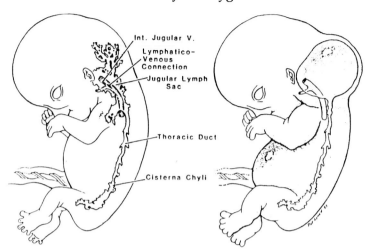

FIG. 14.3. Normal and obstructed lymphatic system. **Left:** The normal fetal lymphatic system. **Right:** Proximal lymphatic obstruction resulting in dilated jugular lymph sacs (posterior cystic hygroma) and generalized lymphedema. (Reprinted from ref. 2 with permission from *The New England Journal of Medicine*, 309, 822–5, 1983.)

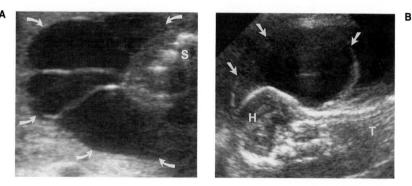

FIG. 14.4. Large posterior cystic hygroma. **A:** A transverse image of the neck at 20 weeks shows a large septated cystic mass (*arrows*) posterior to the cervical spine (S). **B:** A sagittal image of the same fetus shows a large cystic mass (*arrows*) posterior to the head (H) and neck. T, thorax.

A multiseptated cystic mass is present within the soft tissue of the posterior neck. This mass represents accumulated lymphatic fluid in primitive jugular lymph sacs that have failed to drain into the internal jugular vein. Ordinarily additional lymphatic fluid accumulates before reaching the jug-

Posterior Cystic Hygroma (*contd.*)

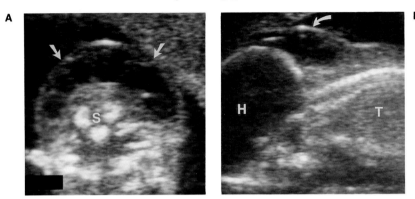

FIG. 14.5. Small posterior cystic hygroma. **A:** A transverse image of the neck at 17 weeks shows a small septated cystic mass (*arrows*) posterior to the cervical spine (S). **B:** A sagittal image of the same fetus shows a small cystic mass (*arrow*) posterior to the head (H) and neck. T, thorax.

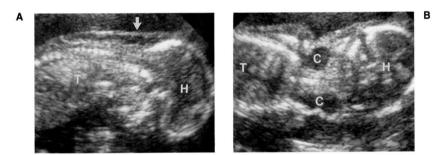

FIG. 14.6. Small mostly lateral posterior cystic hygroma. **A:** A sagittal image of a fetus at 14 weeks shows very little elevation of the skin posterior to the head (H) and neck (*arrow*). T, thorax. **B:** A coronal image of the same fetus shows a symmetric predominantly lateral location of the abnormal posterior cystic mass (C). H, head; T, thorax.

ular lymph sacs and results in generalized marked subcutaneous edema and body cavity fluid. Most fetuses with these findings have chromosomal abnormalities, particularly Turner's syndrome (45,X). Most fetuses with the generalized pattern of abnormalities die before birth. Rarely, findings regress spontaneously. This abnormality should not be confused with an encephalocele or a meningomyelocele.

Cervical Teratoma

A
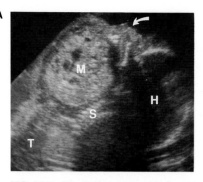

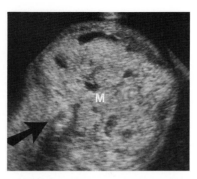
B

FIG. 14.7. Cervical teratoma. **A:** An anterior sagittal image of the head (H), neck, and thorax (T) shows a large, mostly solid mass (M) anterior to the cervical spine (S) and associated displacement of the face (*arrow*) and hyperextension of the neck. (From ref. 3, with permission.) **B:** A transverse image of the neck of the same fetus shows a large, mostly solid mass (M) anterior to the cervical spine (*arrow*).

A solid or complex mass that may originate in the thyroid is present in the anterior neck. Associated hyperextension of the neck may be present. This anomaly often results in death from airway obstruction, although surgical resection may be possible.

Isolated Cystic Hygroma

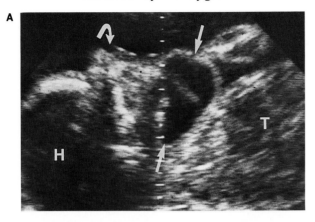

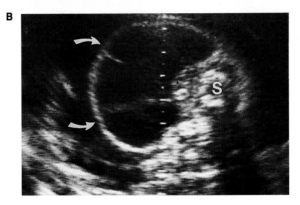

FIG. 14.8. Isolated anterior cystic hygroma. **A:** An anterior sagittal image of the head (H) and thorax (T) at 23 weeks shows a septated cystic mass (*straight arrows*) anterior to the cervical spine and extending toward the face (*curved arrow*). **B:** A transverse image of the same fetus shows a septated cystic mass (*arrows*) anterior to the cervical spine (S).

A multiseptated cystic mass may occur in the soft tissue of the lateral or anterior neck and adjacent portions of the face and thorax. A cystic hygroma in any of these locations is not part of the generalized process described with posterior cystic hygromas. Associated chromosomal abnormalities or additional anomalies are unlikely.

Isolated Cystic Hygroma (*contd.*)

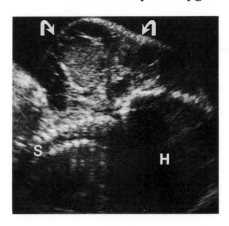

FIG. 14.9. Isolated lateral cystic hygroma. A coronal image of the head and neck at 36 weeks shows a complex mass (*arrows*) lateral to the head (H) and cervical spine (S).

Transient Cervical Cyst

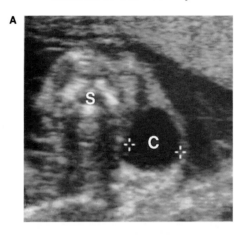

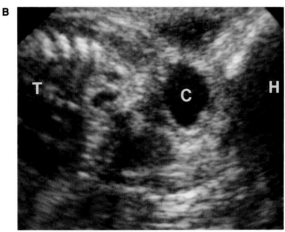

FIG. 14.10. Transient lateral neck cyst. **A:** A posterior transverse image of the neck at 28 weeks shows a small cyst (C) anterior and lateral to the cervical spine (S). **B:** A posterior parasagittal image of the same fetus shows the position of the cyst (C) relative to the head (H) and thorax (T). This cyst resolved on follow-up sonograms. (From ref. 3, with permission.)

Some small cysts in the soft tissue of the neck may be of limited clinical importance and may even resolve spontaneously.

References

1. Benacerraf BR, Barss VA, Laboda LA. A sonographic sign for the detection in the second trimester of the fetus with Down's syndrome. *Am J Obstet Gynecol* 1985;151:1078–9.
2. Chervenak FA, Isaacson G, Blakemore KJ, et al. Fetal cystic hygroma. *N Engl J Med* 1983;309:822–5.
3. Mahony BS, Hegge FN. The face and neck. In: Nyberg DA, Mahony BS, Pretorius DH, eds. *Diagnostic ultrasound of fetal anomalies: text and atlas.* Chicago: Year Book Medical Publishers, 1990;203–61.

Chapter 15

THE SPINE: MID AND LOWER PORTIONS

Scoliosis

A 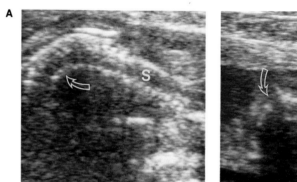 B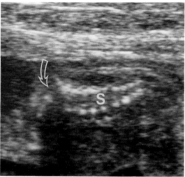

FIG. 15.1 Scoliosis with limb-body wall complex. **A:** An image of the cervical and thoracic spine (S) at 21 weeks shows marked scoliosis (*arrow*) beginning in the lower thoracic spine. **B:** An image of the same fetus in a plane nearly parallel to that of A shows the continuation of the scoliosis (*arrow*) and the position of the lumbosacral spine (S), which is curved nearly 180° from the upper thoracic spine.

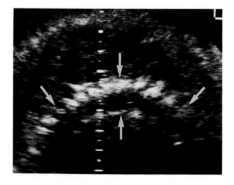

FIG. 15.2. Scoliosis with spinal muscular atrophy. A coronal image of the posterior elements of the spine (*arrows*) at 31 weeks shows marked scoliosis in association with primary spinal cord disease.

Scoliosis (*contd.*)

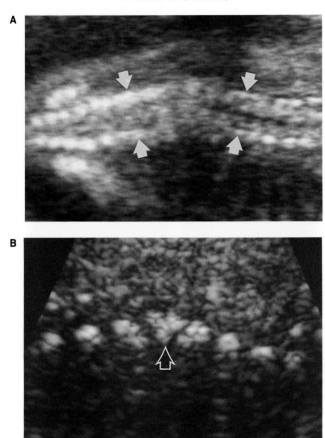

FIG. 15.3. Scoliosis with hemivertebra. **A:** A coronal image of the posterior elements of the spine (*arrows*) at 20 weeks shows mild lumbar scoliosis. **B:** A coronal image of the vertebral bodies shows mild scoliosis in association with an abnormal upper lumbar vertebra (*arrow*) compatible with a hemivertebra.

The spine is curved laterally (scoliosis) and may be rotated and curved anteriorly as well (kyphoscoliosis). These abnormalities may be found as part of a group of anomalies, such as the limb-body wall complex, or as an isolated finding, such as with hemivertebra.

Spina Bifida

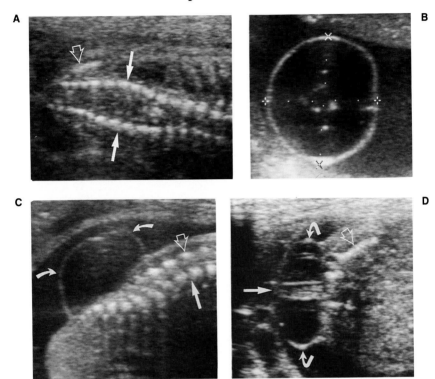

FIG. 15.4. Large meningomyelocele abnormalities. **A:** A coronal image of the lumbosacral spine at 23 weeks shows marked spreading of the posterior elements (*solid arrows*). *Open arrow*, ilium. **B:** A coronal image through the amniotic fluid adjacent to the lumbosacral spine at 26 weeks shows a meningomyelocele sac (*graticules*) 5 cm in diameter. **C:** A sagittal image of the lumbosacral spine at 26 weeks shows a large meningomyelocele sac (*curved arrows*), the vertebral bodies (*straight arrow*), and the posterior elements (*open arrow*), which leave the imaging plane at the level of the sac. **D:** A transverse image of the lower spine of the same fetus shown in C shows a large meningomyelocele sac (*curved arrows*) at the level of the ilium (*open arrow*) and solid tissue (*straight arrow*) within the sac.

With a lumbar or sacral meningomyelocele, the variety most commonly detected by ultrasound, the posterior vertebral arches are split, and neural elements and dura extend into a posterior cystic mass. The position, contents, or integrity of the cystic mass occasionally vary from this pattern. Ordinarily, associated cranial "lemon" and cerebellar "banana" signs are

Spina Bifida (*contd.*)

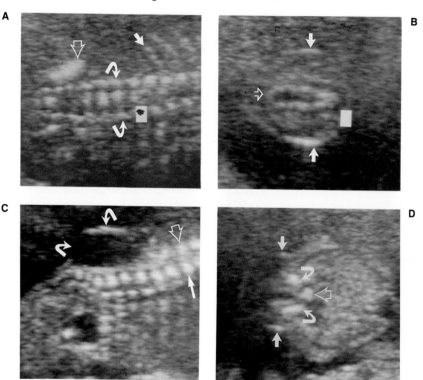

FIG. 15.5. Moderate size meningomyelocele abnormalities. **A:** A coronal image of the lumbosacral spine at 20 weeks shows minimal spreading of the posterior elements (*curved arrows*), the ilium (*open arrow*), the twelfth rib (*straight arrow*), and a cursor on the second lumbar vertebra. **B:** A coronal image through the amniotic fluid adjacent to the lumbosacral spine of the same fetus shows a meningomyelocele sac (*solid arrows*) that contains solid tissue (*open arrow*) and which extends to the second lumbar level according to the cursor location. **C:** A sagittal image of the lumbosacral spine of the same fetus shows a meningomyelocele sac (*curved arrows*) as well as the vertebral bodies (*straight arrow*) and posterior elements (*open arrow*). **D:** A transverse image of the lumbar spine of the same fetus shows the lateral margins of the meningomyelocele sac (*straight arrows*), the vertebral body (*open arrow*), the posterior elements (*curved arrows*), and solid tissue extending from the spinal canal.

present, particularly in the second trimester (see the chapters on the skull and the cerebellum). Sometimes associated hydrocephalus is evident as well (see the chapter on the cerebral ventricles and midline). The more proximal the lesion, the greater the likelihood of severe disability or death.

Spina Bifida (*contd.*)

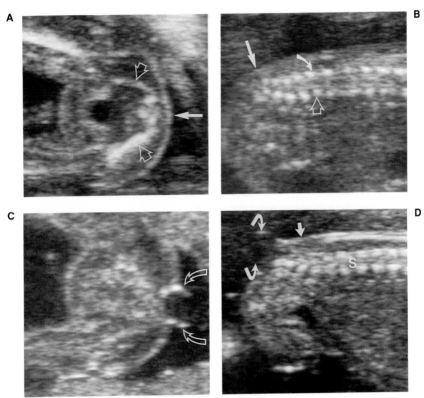

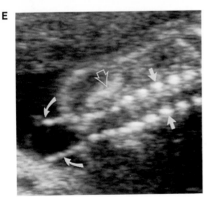

FIG. 15.6. Distal sacral meningomyelocele. **A:** A transverse image of the upper sacrum including the ilia (*open arrows*) and skinline (*closed arrow*) at 20 weeks appears to be unremarkable. **B:** A sagittal image of the skinline (*straight arrow*), posterior elements (*curved arrow*), and vertebral bodies (*open arrow*) of the lumbosacral spine of the same fetus appears to be unremarkable. **C:** A transverse image of the distal sacrum of the same fetus shows a sac (*arrows*) extending through the skinline. **D:** A sagittal image of the lumbosacral spine (S) and skinline (*straight arrow*) in the same fetus that includes the region inferior to the sacrum shows an abnormal sac (*curved arrows*). **E:** A coronal image of the lumbosacral spine of the same fetus that includes the posterior elements (*straight arrows*) and ilia (*open arrow*) as well as the region inferior to the sacrum shows an abnormal sac (*curved arrows*).

Spina Bifida (*contd.*)

A

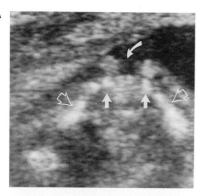

B

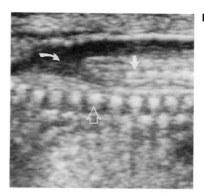

C

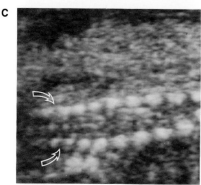

FIG. 15.7. Open spina bifida without a visualized sac. **A:** A transverse image of the sacrum at 18 weeks shows an open defect of the skinline (*curved arrow*) extending to the spinal canal but no overlying sac. *Open arrows*, ilia; *straight arrows*, posterior elements. **B:** A sagittal image of the lumbosacral spine of the same fetus shows the vertebral bodies (*open arrow*), some posterior elements (*straight arrow*), and an open defect of the skinline (*curved arrow*) but no overlying sac. **C:** A coronal image of the lumbosacral spine of the same fetus shows some spreading of the sacral posterior elements (*arrows*), but no sac was evident when the image was moved through the overlying amniotic fluid.

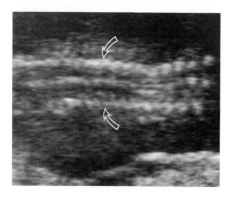

FIG. 15.8. Extensive dysraphism involving much of the spine. A coronal image of the thoracic and lumbar spine at 18 weeks shows abnormal spreading of all visualized posterior elements (*arrows*) in a fetus also found to have anencephaly.

Spina Bifida (*contd.*)

A 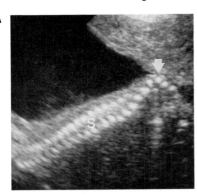 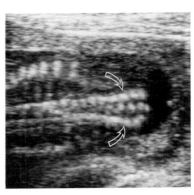 B

FIG.15.9. Spina bifida with marked kyphosis. **A:** A sagittal image of the spine (S) at 19 weeks shows marked lumbar kyphosis (*arrow*) at a level where spina bifida is present on other images. **B:** A coronal image of the spine shows spreading of the posterior elements of the lumbar region (*arrows*) and failure to visualize the remainder of the spine below the level of the kyphosis in this imaging plane.

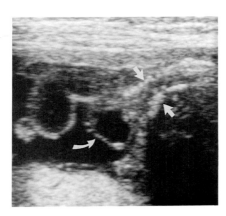

FIG. 15.10. Spina bifida with limb-body wall complex. A coronal image of the spine shows scoliosis, spreading of the posterior elements (*straight arrows*), and abnormal membranes (*curved arrow*).

Sacrococcygeal Teratoma

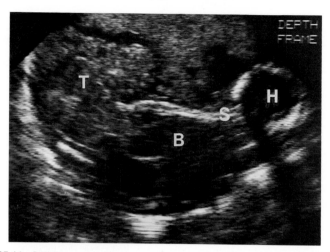

FIG. 15.11. Solid sacrococcygeal teratoma. A posterior sagittal image of the fetus at 21 weeks shows a large solid mass (T) arising from the sacrococcygeal region and located external to the pelvis. H, head; S, spine; B, body.

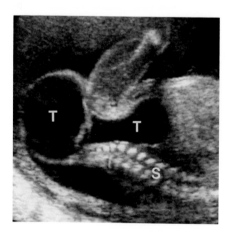

FIG. 15.12. Cystic sacrococcygeal teratoma. An anterior sagittal image of the abdomen and pelvis at 20 weeks shows a large cystic mass (T) arising from the presacral region and extending superiorly within the pelvis and inferiorly external to the pelvis. S, spine.

A solid, cystic, or mixed tumor extends from the presacral region. The tumor may be mostly external, mostly internal, or both internal and external with respect to the perineum. Even though the tumor is often quite large, it is usually benign and surgically resectable.

Incomplete Mineralization

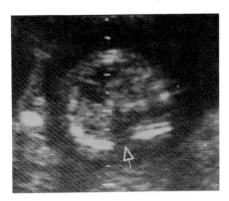

FIG. 15.13. Incomplete mineralization of the spine. A transverse image of the thorax at 16 weeks shows absence of the usual hyperechoic ossification centers of the thoracic spine (*arrow*) in a fetus with achondrogenesis. (From ref. 1, with permission.)

Incomplete mineralization results in reduced or absent ultrasound visualization of the spine. This finding may occur with some kinds of lethal dwarfism, such as achondrogenesis or hypophosphatasia.

Sacral Agenesis and Caudal Regression

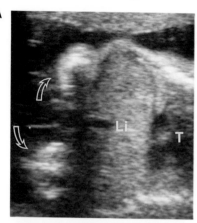

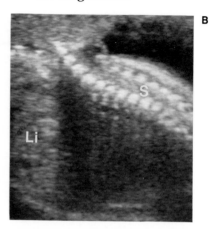

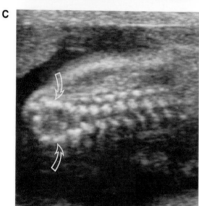

FIG. 15.14. Sacral agenesis. **A:** A coronal image of the thorax (T) and abdomen of a 24-week fetus exposed to maternal diabetes mellitus shows absence of the pelvis resulting in visualization of the flexed lower extremities (*arrows*) immediately inferior to the liver (Li). **B:** A posterior sagittal image of the thorax and abdomen of the same fetus shows the spine (S) ending near the level of the liver (Li). **C:** A posterior coronal image of the spine of the same fetus shows spina bifida (*arrows*) where the lumbar spine ends.

The sacrum and coccyx are absent. With caudal regression, additional abnormalities of the pelvis and lower extremities are present, including hypoplasia, reduction, or fusion (sirenomelia). These anomalies are strongly associated with uncontrolled maternal diabetes mellitus. Associated anomalies of multiple other organ systems are likely to be present as well.

Sacral Agenesis and Caudal Regression (*contd.*)

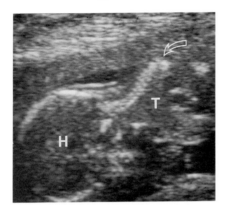

FIG. 15.15. Caudal regression with diabetes mellitus. A posterior sagittal image of the fetus at 15 weeks shows the spine ending (*arrow*) somewhere within the thoracic region in association with uncontrolled maternal diabetes mellitus. T, thorax; H, head. In the same patient, sonography of two subsequent pregnancies also exposed to uncontrolled diabetes mellitus showed a limb reduction abnormality in one and a limb reduction abnormality, hemivertebra, and truncus arteriosus in the other.

Reference

1. Mahony BS, Filly RA, Cooperburg PL. Antenatal sonographic diagnosis of achondrogenesis. *J Ultrasound Med* 1984;3:333–5.

Chapter 16

THE HEART (AND THORAX): NORMAL EXPANDED CARDIAC ANATOMIC EXAMINATION

In fetuses with abnormal cardiac four chamber images or with increased risk for cardiac anatomic abnormalities, an expanded cardiac examination is necessary. The following series of images provides a reasonably complete cardiac anatomic examination. When anatomic abnormalities are present, pulsed Doppler, color Doppler, or M-mode imaging may be required to define the pathophysiology of those abnormalities completely.

Fetal Circulation

In the fetal circulation, umbilical vessels arise from the hypogastric arteries and return to the ductus venosus to carry blood to and from the placenta for oxygenation. In addition, oxygenated blood returning to the right heart bypasses the developing lungs because of shunting through the foramen ovale and through the ductus arteriosus.

In this system both ventricles supply the systemic circulation. Right and left ventricular pressure, size, and muscle thickness are similar as a result. The left ventricle serves the arms and head through the aortic arch. The right ventricle serves the body and legs through the ductus arteriosus and descending aorta.

Many cardiac malformations are well tolerated during fetal life because the right and left sides mix and because the lungs are bypassed. These same malformations become problematic after birth when the right-to-left shunts close and separate systemic and pulmonary circulations with differing pressures are established.

Fetal Circulation (*contd.*)

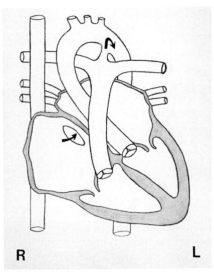

R   L

FIG. 16.1. Drawing of the fetal heart. Illustrated characteristics of the fetal heart include the return of oxygenated blood to the right atrium, shunting of some right atrial blood to the left atrium through the foramen ovale (*lower arrow*), supply of blood to the head and arms from the left ventricle through the aortic arch, supply of blood to the body and legs from the right ventricle by shunting through the patent ductus arteriosus (*upper arrow*), and equal size and wall thickness of the right and left ventricles because both supply the systemic circulation. L, left; R, right. Note the normal crossing pattern and nearly similar size of the aorta and pulmonary artery.

Long Axis Four Chambers and Outflow Tracts

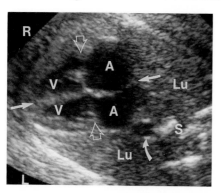

FIG. 16.2. Long axis four chambers. A long axis image of the cardiac four chambers at 28 weeks shows the right and left ventricles and atria (V, A), interventricular and interatrial septa (*straight arrows*), tricuspid and mitral valves (*open arrows*), descending aorta (*curved arrow*), lungs (Lu), and spine (S). R, right; L, left.

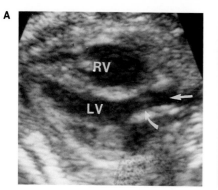
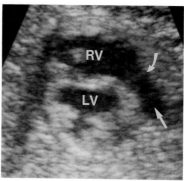

FIG. 16.3. Long axis ventricles and outflow tracts. **A:** A long axis image of the heart at 24 weeks, with the posterior portion of the image angled cephalad compared to Fig. 16.2, shows the right and left ventricles (RV, LV), the aortic valve (*curved arrow*), and the ascending aorta (*straight arrow*), which is continuous with the interventricular septum and crosses the region of the pulmonary artery. **B:** A long axis image of the heart of the same fetus, with the posterior portion of the image angled further cephalad, shows the right and left ventricles (RV, LV), the pulmonary valve (*curved arrow*), and the pulmonary artery (*straight arrow*), which is crossing the region of the aorta.

An oblique transverse real-time image of the thorax is swept through the cardiac four chambers. Subsequently, the posterior portion of this image is swept cephalad from the atria to the crossing outflow tracts. First the aorta is encountered as it exits the left ventricle. Then the pulmonary artery is encountered as it exits the right ventricle.

Short Axis Outflow Tracts and Right Chambers

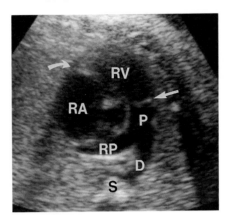

FIG. 16.4. Short axis cardiac image. An oblique transverse image of the thorax shows the right atrium (RA), tricuspid valve (*curved arrow*), right ventricle (RV), pulmonary valve (*straight arrow*), and pulmonary artery (P), surrounding the aortic root as well as the ductal (D) and right (RP) branches but not the left branch of the pulmonary artery. S, spine.

An oblique real-time image of the thorax is swept through the base of the heart. This image shows the right chambers and outflow tract surrounding the left outflow tract.

Parasagittal Aortic and Ductal Arches

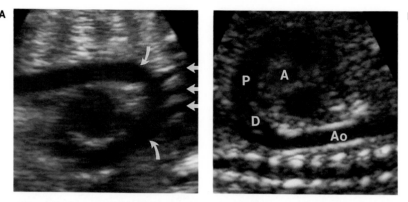

FIG. 16.5. Parasagittal outflow tracts. **A:** A posterior parasagittal image to the left of the spine at 29 weeks shows the aortic arch (*curved arrows*) the neck vessels branching from the arch (*straight arrows*), and the descending aorta. **B:** An anterior parasagittal image closer to the midline at 19 weeks shows the pulmonary artery (P), the ductal arch (D), and the descending aorta (Ao). A, aortic root.

An oblique parasagittal image through the thorax to the left of the spine, which may be obtained either anteriorly or posteriorly, is positioned to include the descending aorta and aortic arch. The image is subsequently positioned to include the descending aorta, ductal arch, and pulmonary artery by assuming a less oblique imaging plane that is closer to the spine.

Pulmonary Veins

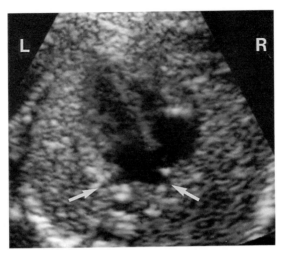

FIG. 16.6. Pulmonary veins. A long axis four chamber image at 16 weeks is angled to show the pulmonary veins (*arrows*) returning to the left atrium. L, left; R, right.

A real-time four chamber image is swept through the left atrium until veins entering its right and left sides are identified.

Superior and Inferior Vena Cava

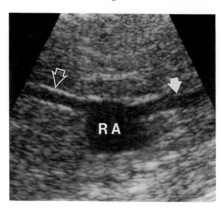

FIG. 16.7. Inferior and superior vena cava. A parasagittal image to the right of the spine at 27 weeks shows the inferior vena cava (*open arrow*) and the superior vena cava (*closed arrow*) entering the right atrium (RA).

A right parasagittal real-time image is swept through the right atrium until veins entering its superior and inferior portions are identified.

Normal Variants or Insignificant Abnormalities

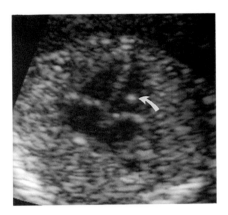

FIG. 16.8. Hyperechoic chordae tendinae. A long axis four chamber image at 18 weeks shows a hyperechoic focus (*arrow*) within the left ventricle near the mitral valve.

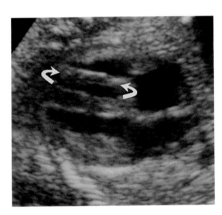

FIG. 16.9. Prominent right ventricular papillary muscle. A long axis four chamber image at 27 weeks shows a prominent papillary muscle (*arrows*) within the right ventricle that appears to extend almost from the apex to the tricuspid valve.

A prominent papillary muscle may be visualized within the right ventricle. The moderator band may be visualized perpendicular to the cardiac long axis within the apical portion of the right ventricle. Occasionally, a hyperechoic focus is present within the chordae tendinae of an atrioventricular valve. This finding appears to have no clinical significance.

Chapter 17

THE HEART (AND THORAX): CARDIAC ABNORMALITIES

Approximately one-third of fetuses who have major anomalies have cardiac anomalies. Most of these anomalies are detectable by prenatal ultrasound before 24 weeks. For many of these fetuses, indications are present for obstetric ultrasound but not for special cardiac examinations. Thus, the potential for the detection of the greatest number of cardiac malformations rests with general obstetric ultrasound rather than with specialized fetal echocardiography. For this potential to be realized, sonographers must be prepared to recognize cardiac malformations and must perform appropriate screening examinations.

Part One: Four Chamber Image Abnormalities

Cardiomegaly and Hydrops

The cardiac chambers are abnormally dilated in association with congestive heart failure. Additional findings of hydrops, which is an excess of body fluid, are likely to be present as well. These findings include some combination of ascites, pleural effusion, pericardial effusion, subcutaneous edema, polyhydramnios, and placental enlargement. Among the many possible etiologies are cardiac arrhythmia, cardiomyopathy, infection, severe anemia from Rh incompatibility, teratomas with high blood flow, and mechanical effects of thoracic masses.

Cardiomegaly and Hydrops (*contd.*)

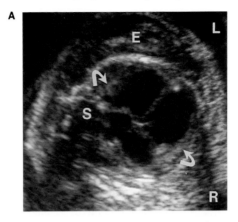

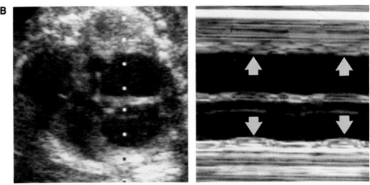

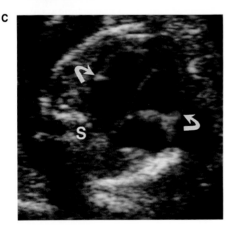

FIG. 17.1. Cardiomegaly with fetal hydrops. **A:** A four chamber cardiac image at 29 weeks shows extreme diffuse cardiomegaly (*arrows*), which was present along with marked subcutaneous edema (E) and marked ascites (not shown). S, spine; R, right; L, left. **B:** An M-mode image of the ventricles of the same fetus shows markedly attenuated ventricular contractions (*arrows*) secondary to cardiomyopathy. **C:** A four chamber cardiac image of another fetus at 24 weeks shows marked cardiomegaly (*arrows*), which was present along with subcutaneous edema and ascites (not shown) secondary to Rh incompatibility. Ventricular wall motion was normal, and all abnormal findings resolved during a series of intrauterine intravascular transfusions. S, spine.

Cardiomegaly and Hydrops (*contd.*)

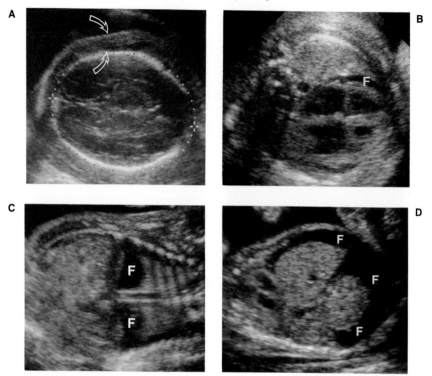

FIG. 17.2. Additional findings with fetal hydrops. **A:** Scalp edema (*arrows*) at 28 weeks with a cervical teratoma. **B:** Pericardial effusion (F) and cardiomegaly at 33 weeks with supraventricular tachycardia. **C:** Pleural effusions (F) at 28 weeks with a cervical teratoma. **D:** Ascites (F) at 25 weeks with anemia from Rh incompatibility.

Ventricular Septal Defect

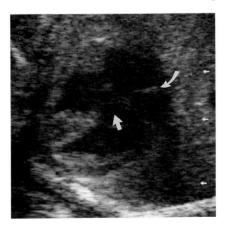

FIG. 17.3. Ventricular septal defect. A four chamber cardiac image at 22 weeks shows a defect in the ventricular septum (*straight arrow*) near the level of the atrioventricular valves in a fetus with multiple anomalies in association with VATERS syndrome. *Curved arrow*, atrial septum.

A defect is present in the interventricular septum, most commonly in the membranous portion near the inlet or outlet valves. This is the most common cardiac anatomic abnormality. It is often present along with other cardiac abnormalities.

Atrioventricular Canal

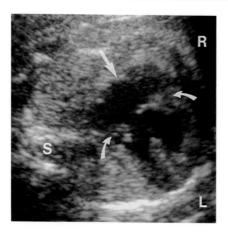

FIG. 17.4. Atrioventricular canal. A four chamber cardiac image at 31 weeks shows contiguous ventricular and atrial septal defects (*straight arrow*) and a common atrioventricular valve (*curved arrows*). S, spine; R, right; L, left.

A complex defect is present in the center of the heart where the plane of the mitral and tricuspid valves crosses the adjacent portions of the ventricular and atrial septa (the region derived from the embryonic endocardial cushion). The defect includes a continuous ventricular and atrial septal defect and abnormalities of adjacent portions of the mitral and tricuspid valves that may result in a common atrioventricular valve. This anomaly is particularly likely to be associated with chromosomal abnormalities, such as trisomies 21, 18, and 13.

Single Ventricle

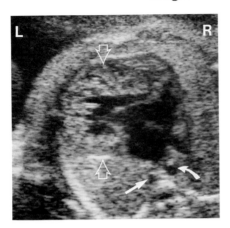

FIG. 17.5. Single ventricle. An image in the usual plane of the cardiac four chambers at 28 weeks shows a large single ventricle (*open arrows*), which is the right ventricle; a single atrioventricular valve; a right-sided aorta (*curved arrow*); and a left-sided continuation of the inferior vena cava (*straight arrow*). L, left; R, right. Abnormal outflow tracts and the atrial septum were defined on other images.

A single ventricular chamber is present. In the double inlet variety, both the mitral and tricuspid valves are present, and the ventricular septum is absent. In the single inlet variety, either the mitral or tricuspid valve is absent (valvular atresia), and only minimal remnants of the associated ventricle are present. As a result, the remaining ventricle becomes a single ventricle served by only one atrioventricular valve.

Ventricular or Atrial Disproportion

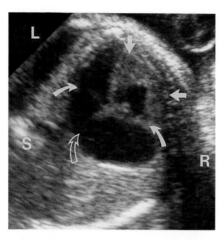

FIG. 17.6. Small right ventricle with muscular hypertrophy. A cardiac four chamber image at 35 weeks shows a small right ventricular cavity, a hypertrophic right ventricular wall (*straight arrows*), and a large right atrium in association with pulmonary stenosis. *Curved closed arrows*, atrioventricular valves; *open arrow*, atrial septum; S, spine; R, right; L, left.

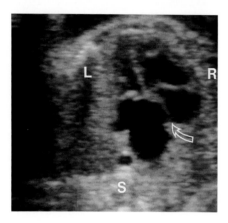

FIG. 17.7. Small left ventricle. A cardiac four chamber image at 32 weeks shows a small left ventricle, a small mitral valve, a large left atrium, and bowing of the atrial septum (*arrow*) to the right rather than to the left in association with aortic stenosis. L, left; R, right; S, spine. (From ref. 1, with permission.)

The normal symmetry between the right and left ventricles and right and left atria is usually lost when valvular abnormalities or some outflow abnormalities are present. Because the four chamber image is used for screening purposes, these findings are often the first clue to the presence of a cardiac abnormality that needs to be further defined.

Ventricular or Atrial Disproportion (*contd.*)

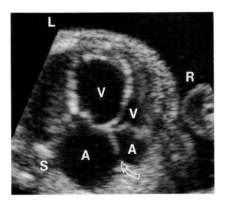

FIG. 17.8. Large left ventricle with endocardial fibroelastosis. A cardiac four chamber image at 29 weeks shows a large left ventricle with a markedly hyperechoic wall, a large left atrium, and bowing of the atrial septum (*arrow*) to the right rather than to the left in association with aortic stenosis. L, left; R, right; V, ventricle; A, atrium; S, spine.

In general, a small (hypoplastic) or absent ventricle is likely to be associated with valvular stenosis or atresia on the same side or with coarctation or interruption of the aorta. Alternatively, a dilated ventricle or hypertrophic or fibrotic ventricular wall may occasionally be present with outflow valvular stenosis. A dilated atrium may be associated with mitral or tricuspid insufficiency. A small atrium may be present with atresia.

Mitral or Tricuspid Valvular Abnormalities

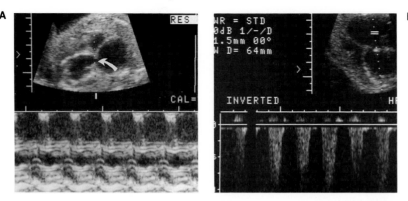

FIG. 17.9. Mitral stenosis. **A:** A modified cardiac long axis image at 29 weeks shows a markedly narrowed mitral valve (*arrow*) between the enlarged left atrium and enlarged hyperechoic left ventricle in association with aortic stenosis. An M-mode image through the mitral valve confirms the marked narrowing and abnormal motion. **B:** Pulse Doppler examination of the enlarged left atrium of the same fetus shows mitral regurgitation.

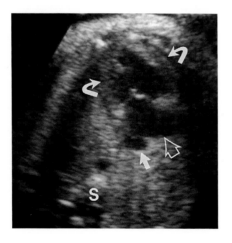

FIG. 17.10. Mitral atresia with single ventricle. An image in the usual plane of the cardiac four chambers at 30 weeks shows a large single ventricle (*curved arrows*), which is the right ventricle; a single atrioventricular valve; a large right atrium (*open arrow*); and a small left atrium (*closed arrow*) in a fetus with absence of the mitral valve, absence of the left ventricle, and a hypoplastic aortic arch.

Mitral or Tricuspid Valvular Abnormalities (*contd.*)

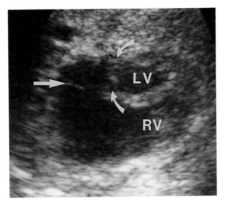

FIG. 17.11. Mitral atresia with hypoplastic left ventricle. A cardiac four chamber image at 33 weeks shows a small partial left ventricle (LV), a small left atrium, and no visualized mitral valve (*curved arrows*) together with the right ventricle (RV) and right atrium. *Straight arrow*, atrial septum.

Possible abnormalities for both atrioventricular valves include atresia (imperforation or absence), stenosis (narrowing), and insufficiency (leakage during closure). In addition, the tricuspid valve may be abnormally positioned near the ventricular apex (Ebstein's anomaly). An atretic valve is closed and thickened or not visualized. A stenotic valve is abnormally small. An insufficient valve is detected by Doppler imaging rather than by anatomic imaging. Associated changes in ventricular and atrial appearance as previously described are likely to be present for all of these valvular abnormalities.

Part Two: Outflow Tract Abnormalities

Aortic or Pulmonic Valvular Abnormalities

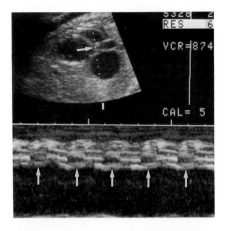

FIG. 17.12. Aortic stenosis. A long axis cardiac image at 29 weeks shows a narrow hyperechoic aortic valve (*upper arrow*) between the dilated left ventricle and the aorta and also shows the right ventricle and the enlarged left atrium. An M-mode image through the aortic valve confirms the hyperechoic appearance and narrow opening of the cusps (*lower arrows*). (See Figs. 17.6 through 17.8 for associated chamber abnormalities with aortic or pulmonary stenosis.)

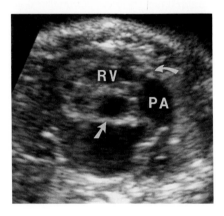

FIG. 17.13. Pulmonary atresia. A short axis cardiac image at 30 weeks shows a small right ventricle (RV), a poorly defined pulmonary valve (*curved arrow*), and the pulmonary artery (PA) adjacent to the aortic root (*straight arrow*).

Possible abnormalities for both outflow valves include atresia and stenosis. An atretic valve is closed or not visualized. A stenotic valve may be small, thickened, or hyperechoic. Doppler imaging may be necessary to differentiate between severe stenosis and atresia. Associated changes in ventricular and atrial appearance as previously described are likely to be present.

Tetralogy of Fallot

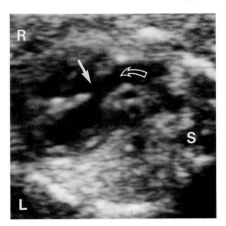

FIG. 17.14. Overriding aorta with tetralogy of Fallot. A long axis image of the ventricles and aorta at 25 weeks shows the aorta (*open arrow*) overriding a ventricular septal defect (*closed arrow*). The pulmonary artery (not shown) was small. R, right; L, left; S, spine.

The aorta overrides the ventricular septum in the region of a ventricular septal defect. The pulmonary valve and pulmonary artery are smaller than the aortic valve and aorta. *In utero* the ventricles may be symmetrical.

Truncus Arteriosus

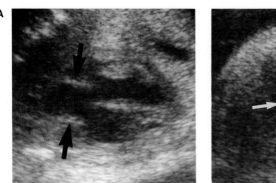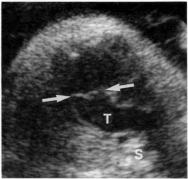

FIG. 17.15. Truncus arteriosus. **A:** A long axis image of the ventricles and outflow region shows a single large outflow vessel (*arrows*) overriding a ventricular septal defect. **B:** A modified short axis image shows a single large outflow valve (*arrows*) and a single large outflow vessel (T). S, spine.

A single large outflow valve and large outflow tract serve both the left and right ventricles because of failure of the embryonic vessel to split into the aorta and pulmonary artery. Usually a ventricular septal defect is present as well, and the truncal valve overrides the ventricular septum. Both the pulmonary arteries and the arteries to the head and neck originate from this truncal vessel, which is contiguous with the aorta.

Complete Transposition

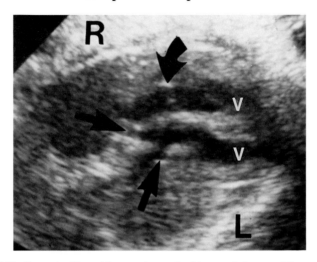

FIG. 17.16. Transposition of the great vessels. A long axis image of the ventricles and outflow regions at 34 weeks shows the outflow vessels leaving the ventricles in a parallel rather than a crossing pattern. The aorta originates in the right ventricle. The pulmonary artery, which is identified by its characteristic branches (*straight arrows*), originates in the left ventricle. *Curved arrow,* aortic valve; R, right; L, left; V, ventricle.

The origins of the outflow tracts are switched so that the aorta originates from the right ventricle and the pulmonary artery originates from the left ventricle. As a result normal crossing of the outflow tracts is not present, and the outflow tracts are parallel to each other in the same plane as the ventricles. Characteristic branching of the aorta and pulmonary artery helps to confirm their identities.

Double Outlet Right Ventricle

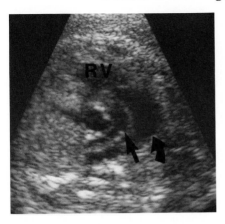

FIG. 17.17. Double outlet right ventricle. A modified short axis cardiac image at 25 weeks shows the larger aorta (*curved arrow*) and the smaller branching pulmonary artery (*straight arrow*) leaving the right ventricle (RV) in the variety of this abnormality with reversed origins and a parallel rather than a crossing pattern.

Both the aorta and the pulmonary artery originate from the right ventricle, usually in association with a ventricular septal defect. The aorta and pulmonary artery may be positioned as usual or transposed with respect to each other. One of the outflow valves may partly override the ventricular septum.

Coarctation of the Aorta

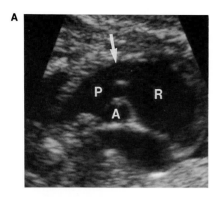

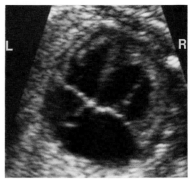

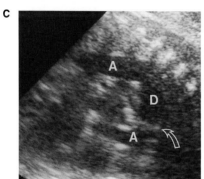

FIG. 17.18. Coarctation of the aorta. **A:** A short axis cardiac image at 31 weeks shows a large pulmonary artery (P) and a small aorta (A). *Arrow*, pulmonary valve; R, right ventricle. **B:** A four chamber cardiac image in the same fetus shows a small left ventricle and left atrium compared to the right ventricle and right atrium. L, left; R, right. **C:** A posterior parasagittal image of the aorta (A) in the same fetus shows inability to visualize much of the aortic arch (*arrow*), although a prominent ductal arch (D) is visualized. On follow-up this finding was found to represent coarctation rather than interruption.

In coarctation a segment of the aortic arch is markedly narrowed, usually in the region of the junction with the ductus arteriosus. In interruption there is actual discontinuity of the aortic arch. Ordinarily, the left ventricle is sufficiently smaller than the right to result in noticeable ventricular disproportion.

Hypoplastic Left Heart Syndrome

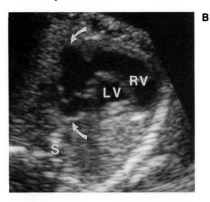

FIG. 17.19. Hypoplastic left heart syndrome. **A:** A posterior sagittal image of the aorta (A) at 30 weeks shows a hypoplastic aortic arch that is markedly narrowed (*arrows*). **B:** A cardiac four chamber image of another fetus at 24 weeks shows a hypoplastic left ventricle compared to the right ventricle (LV, RV) and a hypoplastic left atrium compared to the right atrium (*arrows*). S, spine.

This syndrome includes aortic valvular atresia, mitral valvular atresia or hypoplasia, a small or absent left ventricle, and a hypoplastic aortic arch. Blood flow to the hypoplastic aortic arch, which gives rise to the arteries of the head and neck, is retrograde from the ductus arteriosus.

Part Three: Other Cardiac Abnormalities

Anomalous Pulmonary Venous Return

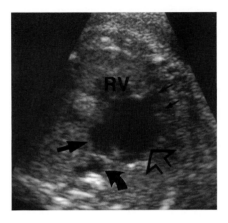

FIG. 17.20. Anomalous pulmonary venous return. An image near the usual plane of the cardiac four chambers at 25 weeks shows pulmonary veins (*small arrows*) returning to a large right atrium (*open arrow*) in a fetus with a right-sided single ventricle (RV), a small left atrium (*straight arrow*), mitral atresia, and abnormal continuation of the inferior vena cava to the left of the aorta (*curved arrow*).

Rather than returning to the left atrium, the pulmonary veins may form a venous confluence posterior to the left atrium and return to some other venous structure. This finding may involve some or all pulmonary veins. It may occur in association with other cardiac malformations or as an isolated finding.

Dextrocardia with Situs Inversus or Situs Ambiguous

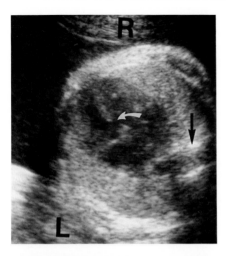

FIG. 17.21. Dextrocardia. A cardiac four chamber image at 35 weeks shows the heart located within the right thorax with its apex directed laterally. A ventricular septal defect (*curved arrow*) is present as well. R, right; L, left; *straight arrow*, spine.

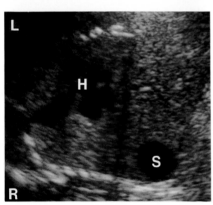

FIG. 17.22. Abnormal heart and right-sided stomach. A coronal image of the thorax and abdomen at 22 weeks shows an abnormal heart (H) located in the left thorax together with gastric fluid (S) located in the right abdomen. L, left; R, right.

Dextrocardia occurs with situs inversus and may occur with situs ambiguous. Situs ambiguous occurs with the asplenia syndrome (bilateral right-sidedness) or the polysplenia syndrome (bilateral left-sidedness). These syndromes may include a right-sided cardiac apex, complex cardiac abnormalities, a right-sided stomach, a central liver, absence of the spleen or bilateral spleens, and duplication, abnormal position, or interruption of the inferior vena cava.

Dextrocardia with Situs Inversus or Situs Ambiguous
(*contd.*)

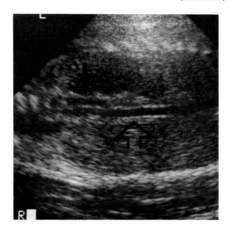

FIG. 17.23. Abnormal heart and malposition of abdominal vessels. A coronal image of the abdomen at 25 weeks shows the inferior vena cava (*closed arrow*) located to the left of the aorta (*open arrow*) in a fetus with cardiosplenic syndrome and complex abnormal heart disease. This finding was confirmed by pulse Doppler examination. L, left; R, right.

Cardiac Rhabdomyoma

A 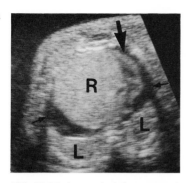 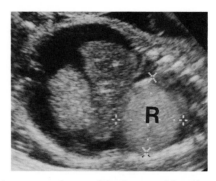 B

FIG. 17.24. Large rhabdomyoma. **A:** A transverse image of the thorax at 29 weeks shows a large solid mass (R) originating in the left ventricle, filling much of the chest, and displacing the remainder of the heart (*large arrow*) to the right. The heart and mass are contained within a pericardial effusion (*small arrows*), and the lungs (L) are displaced posteriorly. **B:** A coronal image of the thorax and abdomen of the same fetus shows the mass (R) filling much of the thorax and shows associated ascites from generalized hydrops.

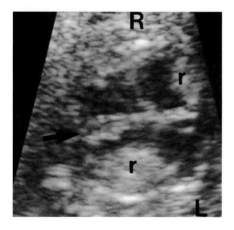

FIG. 17.25. Multiple small rhabdomyomas. A cardiac four chamber image at 32 weeks shows masses (r) originating in the lateral left ventricular wall and in the superior right atrial wall in a fetus later found to have tuberous sclerosis. *Arrow*, ventricular septum; R, right; L, left.

One or more solid masses that originate in the myocardium are present. This finding may be an early sign of tuberous sclerosis.

Pericardial Effusion

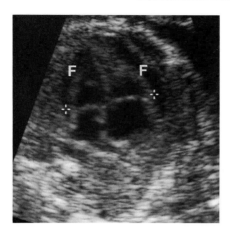

FIG. 17.26. Pericardial effusion. A cardiac four chamber image in a fetus with supraventricular tachycardia and early hydrops shows fluid (F) surrounding the heart (*graticules*).

The heart is surrounded by fluid within the pericardium. This finding usually occurs with generalized fetal hydrops from congestive heart failure or with generalized lymphedema associated with a posterior cystic hygroma.

Arrhythmia

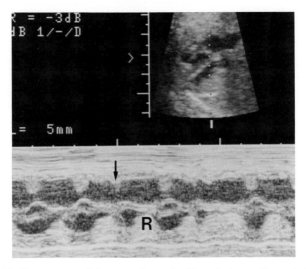

FIG. 17.27. Premature atrial contractions. An M-mode image through the right atrium and left ventricle at 32 weeks shows premature atrial contractions (*arrow*) as well as thickening of the left ventricular wall at the site of a rhabdomyoma (R).

Premature atrial contractions (PACs), supraventricular tachycardia (SVT), complete heart block (CHB), and other arrhythmias may be documented by M-mode imaging. PACs, a relatively common finding, are usually benign and self-limited. Associated bulging of the atrial septum may be present, but more significant associated anomalies are relatively rare. SVT may also be associated with bulging of the atrial septum. If untreated SVT is likely to lead to generalized hydrops and possibly death from congestive heart failure. CHB may be an isolated occurrence or may occur with maternal lupus erythematosus or complex structural cardiac disease.

Arrhythmia (*contd.*)

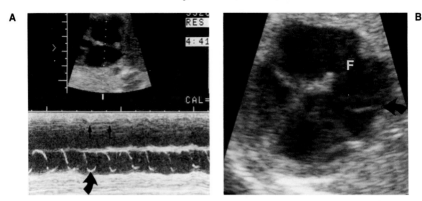

FIG. 17.28. Supraventricular tachycardia. **A:** An M-mode image through the atria at 35 weeks shows atrial tachycardia (*arrows*) at a rate of 220 beats per minute as well as abnormal excursion of the flap of the foramen ovale to the lateral wall of the left atrium. **B:** A cardiac four chamber image of the same fetus shows extension of the atrial septum (*arrow*) from the region of the foramen ovale (F) to the lateral wall of the left atrium. This finding, which has been called an atrial septal aneurysm, may be found with atrial arrhythmias.

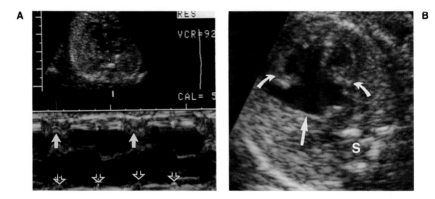

FIG. 17.29. Complete heart block. **A:** An M-mode image through the left ventricle and right atrium at 22 weeks shows an atrial rate (*open arrows*) approximately twice the ventricular rate (*closed arrows*) but dissociated on additional rhythm strips. **B:** A cardiac four chamber image of the same fetus shows a common atrioventricular valve (*curved arrows*) and contiguous ventricular and atrial septal defects (*straight arrow*) typical of an atrioventricular canal. S, spine.

Reference

1. Nyberg DA, Emerson DS. Cardiac malformations. In: Nyberg DA, Mahony BS, Pretorius DH, eds. *Diagnostic ultrasound of fetal anomalies: text and atlas.* Chicago: Year Book Medical Publishers, 1990;300–41.

Chapter 18

THE HEART (AND THORAX): EXTRACARDIAC ABNORMALITIES

Diaphragmatic Hernia

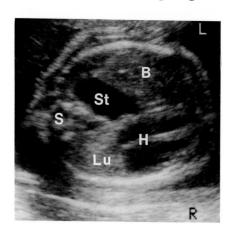

FIG. 18.1. Left diaphragmatic hernia. A transverse image of the thorax at 26 weeks shows herniation of the stomach (St) and bowel (B) into the left thorax with resultant displacement of the heart (H) into the right thorax. S, spine; Lu, lung; L, left; R, right.

Abdominal contents are herniated into the chest through a defect in the diaphragm. The stomach and bowel are most commonly herniated into the left chest, although other organs may be herniated as well, and the heart is displaced into the right chest. The resultant pulmonary compression is likely to result in pulmonary hypoplasia, which contributes to the high mortality rate for this anomaly.

Diaphragmatic Hernia (*contd.*)

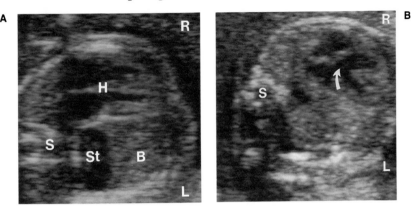

FIG. 18.2. Left diaphragmatic hernia with cardiac abnormality. **A:** A transverse image of the thorax at 22 weeks shows herniation of stomach (St) and bowel (B) into the left thorax and displacement of the heart (H) into the right thorax. S, spine; L, left; R, right. **B:** A slightly different transverse image of the thorax in the same fetus shows a ventricular septal defect (*arrow*) as well as findings of a diaphragmatic hernia. S, spine; L, left; R, right.

Pleural Effusion

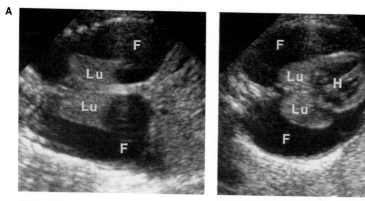

FIG. 18.3. Isolated bilateral pleural effusions. **A:** A coronal image of the thorax at 28 weeks shows bilateral pleural effusions (F) and completely collapsed lungs (Lu). **B:** A transverse image of the thorax of the same fetus shows bilateral pleural effusions (F), completely collapsed lungs (Lu), and the heart (H).

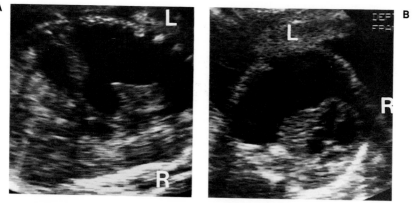

FIG. 18.4. Isolated unilateral pleural effusion. **A:** A coronal image of the thorax at 29 weeks shows a large left pleural effusion and displacement of the collapsed left lung and mediastinum to the right. L, left; R, right. **B:** A transverse image of the thorax of the same fetus shows a large left pleural effusion and displacement of the heart and collapsed lungs to the right. L, left; R, right.

The lung is surrounded by fluid within the pleural space. This may be a unilateral or bilateral isolated finding, such as with idiopathic chylothorax. More commonly, it occurs along with generalized findings of hydrops with congestive heart failure or with a posterior cystic hygroma and generalized lymphedema. Associated pulmonary compression may result in pulmonary hypoplasia if the severity and duration are sufficiently great.

Pulmonary Cystic Adenomatoid Malformation

A

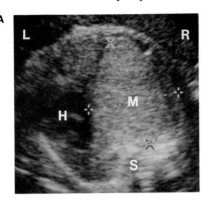 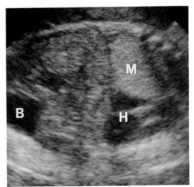

B

FIG. 18.5. Microcystic pulmonary cystic adenomatoid malformation. **A:** A transverse image of the thorax at 40 weeks shows a large hyperechoic mass (M) in the right thorax and displacement of mediastinal contents to the left. H, heart; S, spine; L, left; R, right. **B:** A coronal image of the thorax of the same fetus shows a large hyperechoic mass (M) in the right thorax and displacement of the heart (H) to the extreme left thorax. B, urinary bladder.

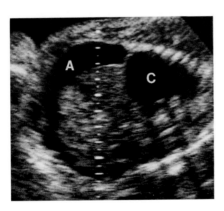

FIG. 18.6. Macrocystic pulmonary cystic adenomatoid malformation. A coronal image of the thorax and abdomen at 32 weeks shows a large cystic mass (C) in the right thorax as well as ascites (A) in the abdomen from associated hydrops.

A pulmonary mass that contains countless small cysts too small to resolve or one or more large or intermediate-sized cysts is present within the chest. If the mass is on the left, the heart may be displaced to the right. Compression of adjacent lung by the mass may cause secondary pulmonary hypoplasia. This mass is a hamartoma that has been classified as macrocystic or microcystic or as types I, II, and III according to descending order of cyst size.

Pulmonary Sequestration

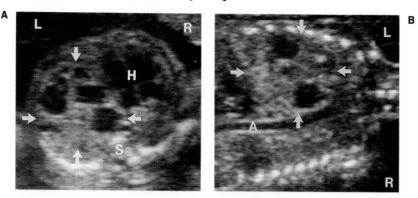

FIG. 18.7. Partly cystic extralobar pulmonary sequestration. **A:** A transverse image of the thorax at 20 weeks shows a large mixed solid and cystic mass (*arrows*) filling the left thorax and displacing the heart (H) to the right. S, spine; L, left; R, right. **B:** A coronal image of the thorax of the same fetus shows a large mixed solid and cystic mass (*arrows*) filling the left thorax and displacing the aorta (A) to the right. L, left; R, right.

A mass of pulmonary parenchyma is isolated from the normal pulmonary parenchyma. Usually the mass has no communication with the normal bronchial tree, and it receives its arterial blood supply from the aorta. It is likely to be located within the chest but may also be located below the diaphragm. It may be solid or may contain cysts. It is classified as extralobar if its pleura is separate from that of the normal parenchyma and as intralobar if it is not. Associated hydrops or pulmonary hypoplasia from compressed lung may be present.

Pulmonary Sequestration (*contd.*)

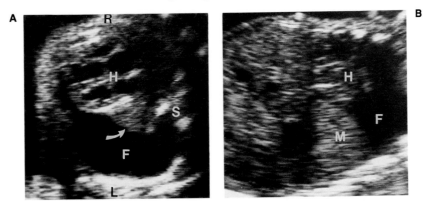

FIG. 18.8. Subphrenic solid extralobar pulmonary sequestration. **A:** A transverse image of the thorax at 27 weeks shows a left pleural effusion (F) displacing the heart (H) and lung (*arrow*) to the right. S, spine; L, left; R, right. **B:** A coronal image of the thorax and abdomen of the same fetus shows a left pleural effusion (F), displacement of the heart (H) to the right thorax, and a left subphrenic solid mass (M), which was found to be extralobar pulmonary sequestration.

Deformed Ribs

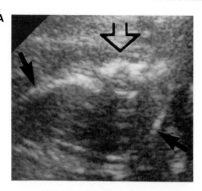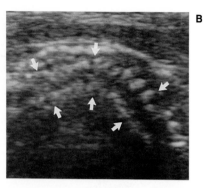

FIG. 18.9. Deformed ribs with limb-body wall complex. **A:** A transverse image of the thorax at 21 weeks shows bowing of the ribs to be abnormally acute on one side and abnormally obtuse on the other (*closed arrows*). *Open arrow*, spine. **B:** A coronal image of the spine of the same fetus shows associated scoliosis (*arrows*).

The configuration of the rib cage may be markedly distorted when scoliosis is present, particularly in association with the limb-body wall complex. The rib cage may be markedly narrowed and the ribs may be abnormally shortened or fractured in association with some varieties of lethal dwarfism.

Deformed Ribs (*contd.*)

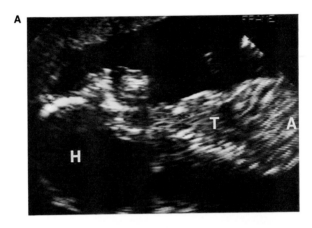

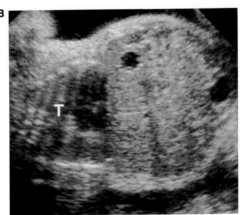

FIG. 18.10. Narrow thorax with lethal dwarfism. **A:** A sagittal image of the head and body at 25 weeks shows anteroposterior narrowing of the thorax (T) of a fetus with thanatophoric dwarfism. H, head; A, abdomen. **B:** A coronal image of the thorax and abdomen at 34 weeks shows transverse narrowing of the thorax (T) in a fetus with homozygous achondroplasia.

Subcutaneous Edema

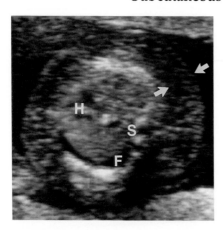

FIG. 18.11. Thoracic subcutaneous edema with cystic hygroma. A transverse image of the thorax at 16 weeks shows marked thickening of the subcutaneous region (*arrows*) as well as a small pleural effusion (F) in association with a posterior cystic hygroma and generalized lymphedema. S, spine; H, heart.

The subcutaneous tissue of the thorax is abnormally thickened because of edema with hydrops from congestive heart failure or with a posterior cystic hygroma and generalized lymphedema.

Chapter 19

GASTRIC FLUID (AND ABDOMEN)

Early Second Trimester Hyperechoic Bowel

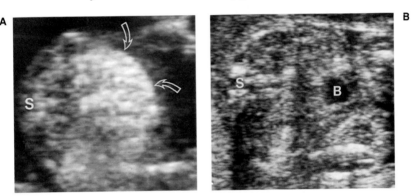

FIG. 19.1. Hyperechoic small bowel. **A:** A transverse image of the abdomen at 16 weeks shows a region of hyperechoic small bowel (*arrows*). S, spine. **B:** A transverse image of the abdomen of the same fetus at 22 weeks shows resolution of the hyperechoic small bowel. S, spine; B, urinary bladder.

A diffusely hyperechoic appearance of small bowel may be present in the early second trimester. Although originally reported to be associated with cystic fibrosis, this finding is likely to be normal when no associated calcifications or fluid collections are present and when resolution occurs on follow-up sonograms.

Esophageal Atresia

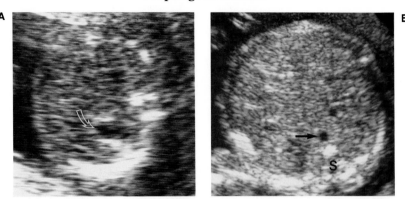

FIG. 19.2. Esophageal atresia with tracheoesophageal fistula. **A:** A transverse image of the abdomen at 17 weeks shows well-defined gastric fluid (*arrow*). **B:** A transverse image of the abdomen of the same fetus at 22 weeks shows no well-defined gastric fluid. A few weeks later, polyhydramnios was present as well. *Arrow*, aorta; S, spine.

A portion of the esophagus is missing. After 24 weeks abnormal swallowing results in polyhydramnios in a majority of cases, but gastric fluid is reduced or absent in only a minority because of the frequent association with tracheoesophageal fistula. Abnormal swallowing from facial or central nervous system disorders may result in similar findings.

Duodenal Atresia

A

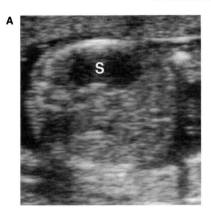

B

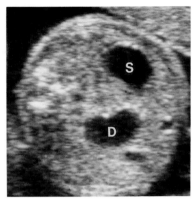

C

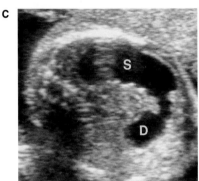

FIG. 19.3. Duodenal atresia. **A:** A transverse image of the abdomen at 20 weeks shows only well-defined gastric fluid (S). **B:** A transverse image of the abdomen of the same fetus at 26 weeks shows a double bubble of fluid within the stomach (S) and within the duodenum (D). Polyhydramnios was present as well. **C:** A slightly oblique transverse image of the abdomen of the same fetus shows continuity of fluid between the stomach (S) and the duodenum (D) and confirms that the right-sided fluid has duodenal origin.

A portion of the duodenum is imperforate. After 24 weeks a "double bubble" from fluid in the abnormally dilated proximal duodenum together with gastric fluid is present. Polyhydramnios from reduced ingestion of amniotic fluid is likely to be present as well. Associated trisomy 21 is present in about one-third of cases.

Duodenal Atresia (*contd.*)

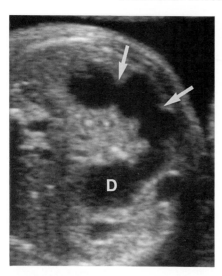

FIG. 19.4. Prominent peristalsis with bowel obstruction. An oblique transverse image of the abdomen at 30 weeks shows fluid in the stomach and in an obstructed duodenum (D) as well as prominent peristaltic waves (*arrows*) in the stomach.

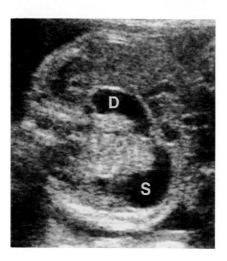

FIG. 19.5. Double bubble with annular pancreas. An oblique transverse image of the abdomen at 32 weeks shows fluid in the stomach (S) and in an obstructed duodenum (D) in association with an annular pancreas.

Jejunal or Ileal Atresia

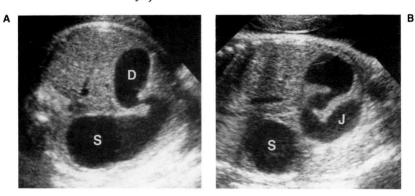

FIG. 19.6. High jejunal atresia. **A:** A transverse image of the abdomen at 33 weeks shows fluid in a dilated stomach (S) and duodenum (D). **B:** A coronal image of the abdomen of the same fetus shows fluid in dilated loops of proximal jejunum (J) as well as in the stomach (S).

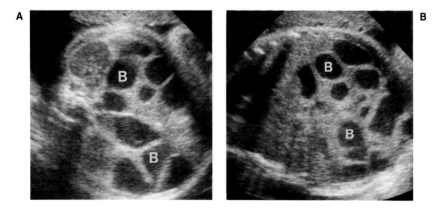

FIG. 19.7. Mid small bowel atresia. **A, B:** Transverse and coronal images of the abdomen at 36 weeks show many dilated fluid-filled loops of small bowel (B).

A portion of the jejunum or ileum is imperforate. After 24 weeks small bowel proximal to the obstruction is abnormally dilated. Polyhydramnios from reduced ingestion of amniotic fluid may be present as well, but it is less likely in distal obstruction.

Meconium Peritonitis

A

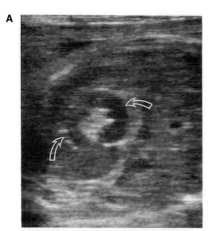

B

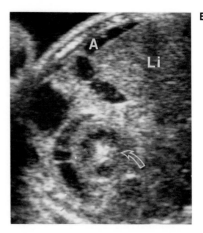

C

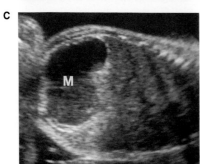

FIG. 19.8. Evolution of a meconium cyst. **A:** An image of the abdomen at 29 weeks shows a single loop of abnormally dilated bowel (*arrows*) with volvulus. **B:** An image of the abdomen at 30 weeks shows the same loop of abnormally dilated bowel (*arrow*). It also shows mild ascites (A) at the liver (Li) margin and elsewhere in the abdomen compatible with bowel perforation. **C:** A coronal image of the abdomen at 32 weeks shows a large cystic mass (M) with a hyperechoic wall and echogenic contents that represents a walled-off bowel perforation.

Bowel perforation that arises spontaneously or in association with any obstructing lesion results in leakage of bowel contents into the peritoneal cavity. The intense chemical peritonitis that follows may produce calcifications, ascites, or a walled-off cystic mass (meconium cyst). Cystic fibrosis may be a predisposing factor in a relatively small minority of cases.

Meconium Peritonitis (*contd.*)

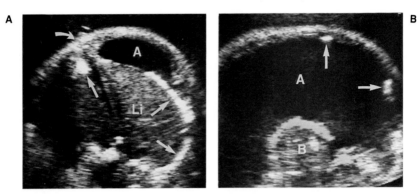

FIG. 19.9. Generalized meconium peritonitis. **A:** A transverse image of the abdomen at the level of the liver (Li) at 36 weeks shows ascites (A), intense calcification at the liver margin (*straight arrows*), and adhesion of the liver margin to the abdominal wall (*curved arrow*). **B:** A transverse image of the abdomen of the same fetus at the level of the small bowel (B) shows marked ascites (A), focal calcifications (*arrows*), and a rind of calcification surrounding the small bowel.

Ascites

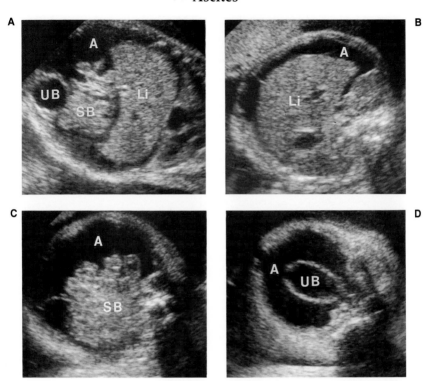

FIG. 19.10. Ascites with generalized hydrops. **A:** A coronal image of the abdomen at 34 weeks shows ascites (A) surrounding the liver (Li), small bowel (SB), and urinary bladder (UB). **B, C, D:** Transverse images of the abdomen of the same fetus show ascites (A) at the level of the liver (Li), small bowel (SB), and urinary bladder (UB).

The abdominal contents are surrounded by free fluid within the peritoneal cavity. This finding usually occurs with generalized hydrops from congestive heart failure or with generalized lymphedema with a posterior cystic hygroma. It may also occur as an isolated finding, such as with meconium peritonitis.

Hepatic Calcifications

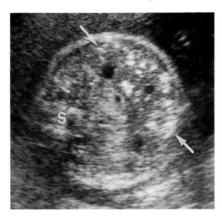

FIG. 19.11. Hepatic calcifications with cytomegalovirus. A transverse image of the abdomen at 28 weeks in a fetus infected with cytomegalovirus shows multiple calcifications throughout the liver (*arrows*). S, spine.

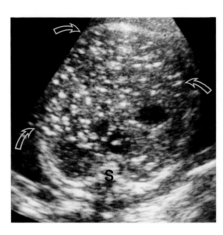

FIG. 19.12. Hepatic calcifications with varicella. A transverse image of the abdomen at 30 weeks in a fetus with varicella infection shows many small calcifications throughout the liver (*arrows*). S, spine.

Focal calcifications are present throughout the liver. This finding is strongly associated with fetal infection, such as with cytomegalovirus or varicella.

Abdominal Cystic Mass

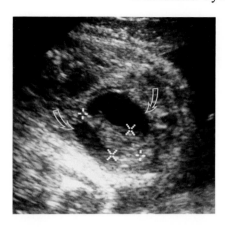

FIG. 19.13. Ovarian cyst. A transverse image of the abdomen of a female fetus at 32 weeks shows a complex cystic mass (*arrows*) that contains internal solid material compatible with thrombus (*graticules*).

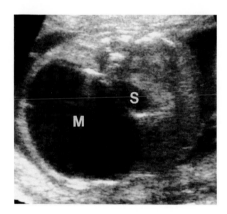

FIG. 19.14. Large abdominal cystic mass. A transverse image of the abdomen at 18 weeks shows a large cystic mass (M) that is displacing the stomach (S) medially. This mass was found to be fetus in fetu, which is similar to a teratoma, on postmortem examination.

A pelvic or abdominal cystic mass in a female fetus is likely to be an ovarian cyst. An ovarian cyst may contain septa or echogenic material, particularly in association with hemorrhage or torsion. Cystic masses of other origin, such as duplication cysts, mesenteric cysts, or teratomas, are less common. Cystic masses should be differentiated from dilated bowel or urinary tract structures that may have a similar appearance.

Abdominal Solid Mass

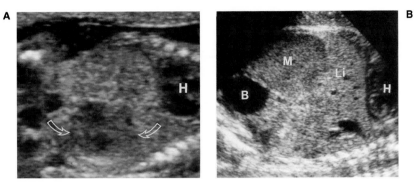

FIG. 19.15. Solid hepatic mass. **A:** A coronal image of the abdomen at 22 weeks shows a large hypoechoic mass (*arrows*) near the liver. H, heart. **B:** A coronal image of the abdomen of the same fetus at 35 weeks shows a large hypoechoic mass (M) originating in the liver (Li). H, heart; B, urinary bladder. The mass was found to be a hemangioendothelioma (from ref. 1, with permission.).

Solid abdominal masses are rarely encountered prenatally. When present, they may originate from the liver as well as from other abdominal structures.

Situs Abnormalities

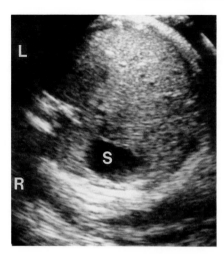

FIG. 19.16. Situs inversus. A transverse image of the abdomen at 34 weeks shows gastric fluid (S) on the right side. R, right; L, left. Other abdominal organs and the heart were reversed as well.

With situs inversus and with some cases of situs ambiguous (asplenia or polysplenia syndromes), the stomach is located within the right side of the abdomen. When this finding is present, evaluation of the position of the aorta, inferior vena cava, liver, gall bladder, spleen, and heart as well as the structure of the heart will help to define the nature of the situs abnormality (see the chapter on cardiac abnormalities).

Subcutaneous Edema

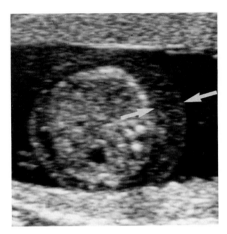

FIG. 19.17. Abdominal subcutaneous edema with cystic hygroma. A transverse image of the abdomen at 16 weeks shows marked thickening of the subcutaneous region (*arrows*) in association with a posterior cystic hygroma and generalized lymphedema.

The subcutaneous tissue of the abdominal wall is abnormally thickened because of edema from hydrops with congestive heart failure or from generalized lymphedema with a posterior cystic hygroma.

Reference

1. Nyberg DA. Intra-abdominal abnormalities. In: Nyberg DA, Mahoney BS, Pretorius DH, eds. *Diagnostic ultrasound of fetal anomalies: text and atlas.* Chicago: Year Book Medical Publishers, 1990;342–94.

Chapter 20

THE KIDNEYS

With hydronephrosis, the width of the fluid in the renal pelvis is abnormally increased. According to one source, renal pelvic widths of less than 5 mm or less than one-third the renal width are normal, and renal pelvic widths of more than 9 mm or more than one-half the renal width usually indicate significant hydronephrosis. Intermediate widths are usually normal but may require follow-up (1). Another source recommends postnatal follow-up for pelvic widths of 4 mm before 20 weeks, 5 mm at 20 to 26 weeks, 6 mm at 27 to 35 weeks, and 7 mm at more than 35 weeks (2).

Associated findings such as caliectasis, hydroureter, or abnormal parenchyma also help to indicate the presence of significant hydronephrosis. Marked dilatation of the renal pelvis and calyces and marked thinning of the renal parenchyma indicate the presence of severe hydronephrosis.

Ureteropelvic Junction (UPJ) Obstruction

A 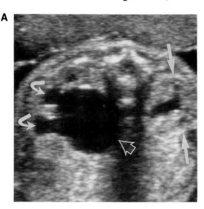 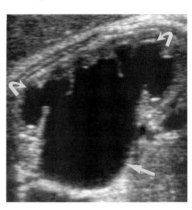 B

FIG. 20.1. Hydronephrosis with UPJ obstruction. **A:** A posterior transverse image of the kidneys at 30 weeks shows no hydronephrosis of one kidney (*straight arrows*) but moderate hydronephrosis of the other kidney, including pyelectasis (*open arrow*), caliectasis (*curved arrows*), and intact surrounding renal parenchyma. **B:** A coronal image of the abnormal kidney of the same fetus at 36 weeks shows prominent pyelectasis (*straight arrow*), caliectasis (*curved arrows*), some remaining renal parenchyma, and no apparent hydroureter.

Unilateral or bilateral hydronephrosis is present in association with obstruction at the junction of the renal pelvis and ureter. The ureters and urinary bladder are unremarkable.

Ureterovesicular Junction (UVJ) Obstruction

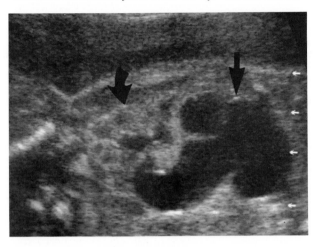

FIG. 20.2. Hydronephrosis with duplex kidney. A coronal image of a duplex kidney at 23 weeks shows an upper pole hydronephrotic sac (*straight arrow*), the proximal portion of contiguous hydroureter, and a nonhydronephrotic lower pole (*curved arrow*).

A duplex renal collecting system may be a cause of ureterovesicular junction obstruction. Hydronephrosis may be present in one portion of a duplex kidney, usually the upper portion, in association with hydroureter and an ectopic ureterocele where the duplex ureter enters the urinary bladder.

Ureterovesicular Reflux

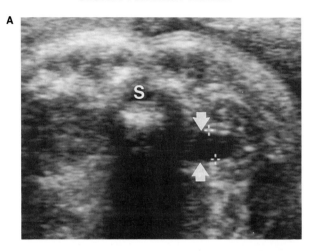

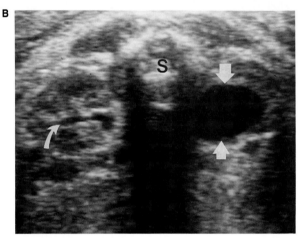

FIG. 20.3. Hydronephrosis with UVJ reflux. **A:** A transverse image of the kidneys at 33 weeks shows mild left pyelectasis (*arrows*). S, spine, **B:** A similar image a few seconds later shows considerably increased size of the left renal pelvis (*straight arrows*) and a normal volume of fluid in the right renal pelvis (*curved arrow*). S, spine. A postnatal voiding cystogram showed marked left UVJ reflux.

Hydronephrosis may be present in association with reflux of urine from the bladder into the ureters and renal pelvis through an incompetent ureterovesical junction. Hydroureter may be present as well.

Urinary Bladder Outlet Obstruction

A
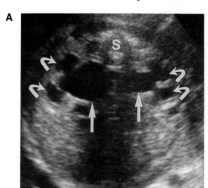

B
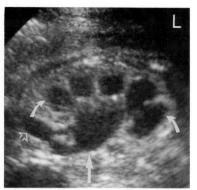

C
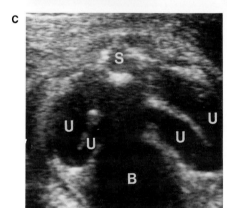

FIG. 20.4. Hydronephrosis with bladder outlet obstruction. **A:** A transverse image of the kidneys at 26 weeks shows bilateral pyelectasis (*straight arrows*) and caliectasis (*curved arrows*) consistent with moderate hydronephrosis. S, spine. **B:** A coronal image of the left kidney shows caliectasis (*curved arrows*), pyelectasis (*straight arrow*), and contiguous hydroureter (*open arrow*). L, left. **C:** A posterior transverse image of the abdomen of a similar fetus at 32 weeks shows bilateral hydroureter (U). S, spine; B, bladder.

Hydronephrosis is present bilaterally in association with obstructed outflow from the urinary bladder, usually from posterior urethral valves in a male fetus. Bilateral hydroureter, urinary bladder dilatation or wall thickening, and dilatation of the posterior urethra are ordinarily present as well. In severe cases renal dysplasia, urinoma formation, urine ascites, and oligohydramnios may be present.

Dysplastic Kidneys

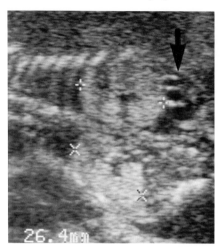

FIG. 20.5. Renal dysplasia with bladder outlet obstruction. A coronal image of the thorax and abdomen at 22 weeks shows bilaterally enlarged kidneys with diffusely hyperechoic parenchyma (*graticules*) as well as hydroureter (*arrow*). Oligohydramnios is present as well.

Severe urinary bladder outlet obstruction may be associated with renal parenchymal changes that result in abnormally small or large kidneys, hyperechoic kidneys, or many renal cysts. These changes may occur without associated hydronephrosis. Together with oligohydramnios, they indicate a poor prognosis.

Renal Agenesis

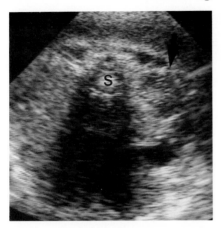

FIG. 20.6. Unilateral renal agenesis. A posterior transverse image of the regions of the kidneys at 35 weeks shows a visualized kidney in one renal fossa (*arrow*) but not in the other. S, spine.

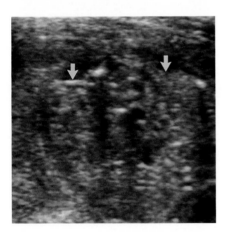

FIG. 20.7. Bilateral renal agenesis. A posterior transverse image of the regions of the kidneys at 23 weeks shows marked oligohydramnios and no visualized kidney in either renal fossa (*arrows*).

One or both kidneys are absent. If only one kidney is absent, other related findings are unlikely if the remaining kidney is normal. If both kidneys are absent, the urinary bladder is not visualized, and profound oligohydramnios is present. The fetus has Potter's syndrome at birth, which includes facial deformity, contractures, and death from pulmonary hypoplasia as a result of oligohydramnios.

Multicystic Kidneys

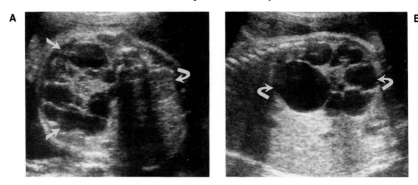

FIG. 20.8. Unilateral multicystic kidney. **A:** A posterior transverse image of the kidneys at 29 weeks shows a normal kidney (*curved arrow*) in one renal fossa and a multicystic mass (*straight arrows*) without the pattern of the renal pelvis and calyces in the other renal fossa. **B:** A coronal image of the same fetus shows the random multicystic appearance of the parenchyma of the abnormal kidney (*arrows*).

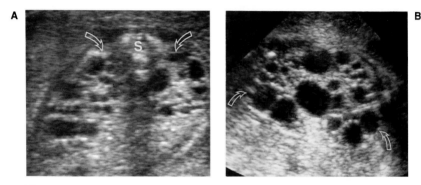

FIG. 20.9. Bilateral multicystic kidney. **A:** A posterior transverse image of the kidneys shows an abnormal random multicystic appearance of both kidneys (*arrows*) as well as marked oligohydramnios. S, spine. **B:** A posterior sagittal image of one of the abnormal kidneys of the same fetus shows the random multicystic appearance of the parenchyma of that kidney (*arrows*).

One or both kidneys are enlarged because of extensive parenchymal replacement by cysts of variable sizes. Affected kidneys are nonfunctional. If both kidneys are affected, the urinary bladder is not visualized, and profound oligohydramnios is present. The fetus has Potter's syndrome at birth, which includes facial deformity, contractures, and death from pulmonary hypoplasia as a result of oligohydramnios. This abnormality is differentiated from hydronephrosis by the lack of an identifiable central pelvis and by the lack of communication between cysts.

Isolated Renal Cysts

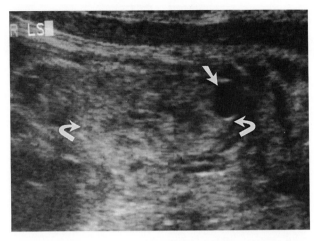

FIG. 20.10. Isolated renal cyst. A sagittal image of a kidney (*curved arrows*) at 35 weeks shows an isolated cyst (*straight arrow*). On postnatal follow-up, the kidneys were otherwise unremarkable, and there was no family history of renal disease.

Rarely, one or more isolated renal cysts are present. These cysts may be an indication of dysplasia or adult polycystic disease. They should be differentiated from urinoma formation with hydronephrosis.

Paranephric Urinoma

A
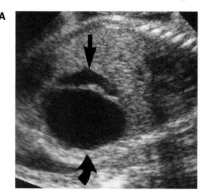

B
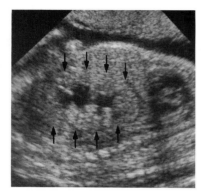

C
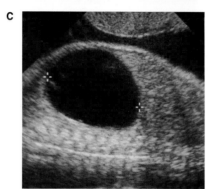

FIG. 20.11. Paranephric urinoma. **A:** A coronal image of a fetus with UPJ obstruction at 31 weeks shows a medial dilated renal pelvis (*straight arrow*) and a larger lateral urinoma (*curved arrow*) from rupture of the renal collecting system. **B:** A midsagittal image of the same fetus shows a kidney (*arrows*) that is markedly flattened against the large urinoma, which is not shown in this imaging plane. **C:** A parasagittal image of the same fetus shows the large urinoma (*graticules*) located immediately lateral to the flattened kidney.

A loculated retroperitoneal fluid collection is present in the region of the kidney. This finding is the result of rupture of a renal collecting system in association with obstructive hydronephrosis.

Polycystic Kidneys

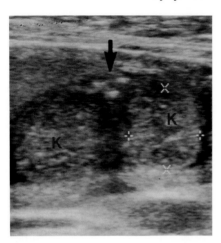

FIG. 20.12. Polycystic kidneys. A posterior transverse image of the abdomen at 17 weeks in a fetus with Meckel-Gruber syndrome shows kidneys (K) that are bilaterally markedly enlarged and hyperechoic because of many small parenchymal cysts too small to resolve individually. *Arrow,* spine.

In the autosomal recessive infantile variety, the kidneys are enlarged because of extensive replacement of their parenchyma by many small cysts, which ordinarily result in a hyperechoic rather than a multicystic appearance. In the autosomal dominant adult variety, enlarged hyperechoic kidneys or kidneys containing cysts may be encountered, but the kidneys may also appear to be normal. With Meckel-Gruber syndrome, the kidneys may be enlarged and hyperechoic because of many very small cysts.

Abnormally Large Kidneys

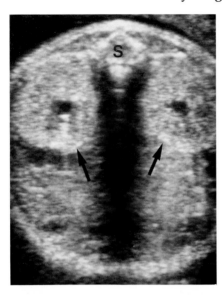

FIG. 20.13. Large kidneys of uncertain etiology. A posterior transverse image of the abdomen at 35 weeks shows abnormally large, hyperechoic kidneys (*arrows*). S, spine. Short-term postnatal follow-up showed normal renal function.

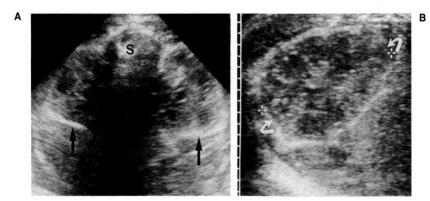

FIG. 20.14. Large kidneys with Beckwith-Wiedemann syndrome. **A:** A posterior transverse image of the kidneys (*arrows*) at 37 weeks shows that they are subjectively large relative to the abdomen. S, spine. **B:** A parasagittal image of one of the kidneys (*arrows*, *graticules*) in the same fetus shows that it is abnormally enlarged to a length of 6.4 cm.

The kidneys may be abnormally large with some syndromes or diseases, such as Beckwith-Wiedemann syndrome or renal vein thrombosis, as well as with multicystic, polycystic, and dysplastic disease.

Ectopia

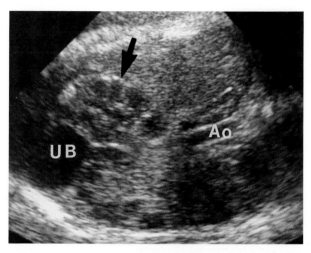

FIG. 20.15. Pelvic kidney. A coronal image of a fetus at 36 weeks with one kidney not visualized in the renal fossa shows a kidney (*arrow*) located in the pelvis adjacent to the urinary bladder (UB). Ao, aorta.

A kidney that is not present in its usual position in the renal fossa may be located within the pelvis or fused with the contralateral kidney. When a kidney is not visualized in the renal fossa, renal ectopia is differentiated from unilateral renal agenesis by a careful search of possible ectopic sites.

References

1. Arger PH, Coleman BG, Mintz MC. Routine fetal genitourinary tract screening. *Radiology* 1985;156:485–9.
2. Corteville JE, Gray DL, Crane JP. Congenital hydronephrosis: correlation of fetal sonographic findings with infant outcomes. *J Ultrasound Med* 1990; 9:S1–S124.

Chapter 21

THE UMBILICAL CORD INSERTION SITE

Normal Bowel Migration

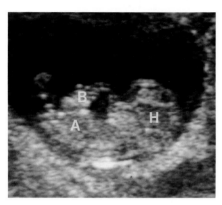

FIG. 21.1. Normal bowel migration. A sagittal image of an embryo at 10 weeks shows bowel (B) within the umbilical cord, a normal finding at this gestational age. H, head; A, abdomen.

Bowel is transiently present within the umbilical cord of the embryo at 8 to 10 weeks and may be present until 12 weeks. This normal finding should not be mistaken for a body wall defect.

Gastroschisis

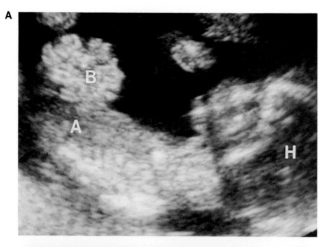

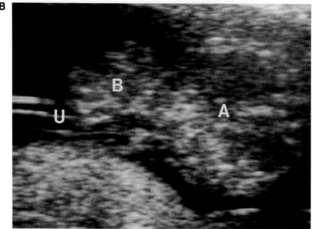

FIG. 21.2. Gastroschisis. **A, B:** Anterior sagittal and transverse images at 18 weeks show a clump of bowel (B), which is eviscerated into the amniotic fluid through a body wall defect to the right of the umbilical cord (U) and which has an irregular margin because of the lack of a covering membrane. H, head; A, abdomen.

Bowel extends through a paraumbilical body wall defect, which is usually right-sided, into the amniotic fluid. The eviscerated bowel is located adjacent to rather than within the umbilical cord. No covering membrane is present. Chromosomal abnormalities and associated anomalies are unlikely.

Gastroschisis (*contd.*)

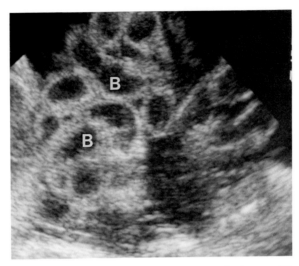

FIG. 21.3. Dilated bowel with gastroschisis near term. An image of the eviscerated bowel (B) of the fetus shown in Fig. 21.2 at 38 weeks shows that the bowel has become dilated, fluid filled, and thick walled because of irritation by exposure to amniotic fluid.

Omphalocele

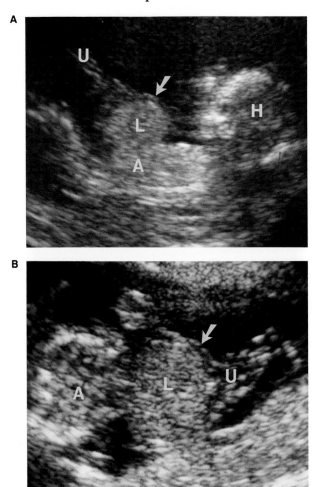

FIG. 21.4. Omphalocele containing liver. **A, B:** Sagittal and transverse images of the fetus at 15 weeks show liver (L) within an omphalocele that is contained by a membrane (*arrow*) and located within the base of the umbilical cord (U). H, head; A, abdomen.

Abdominal contents are herniated into the base of the umbilical cord. The herniated contents, which may include some combination of liver, bowel, ascites, and sometimes other organs, are contained within a membrane. Chromosomal abnormalities and associated anomalies are likely; hence, differentiation from gastroschisis is important.

Omphalocele (*contd.*)

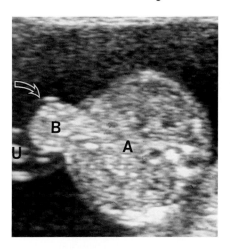

FIG. 21.5. Small omphalocele containing bowel. A transverse image of the abdomen (A) of an18-week fetus with Beckwith-Wiedemann syndrome shows a small omphalocele that contains only bowel (B), which is covered by a membrane (*arrow*) and located within the base of the umbilical cord (U).

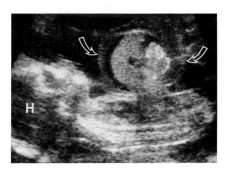

FIG. 21.6. Omphalocele containing liver and bowel. A sagittal image of the fetus at 20 weeks shows the membrane of an omphalocele (*arrows*) surrounding liver and bowel. H, head.

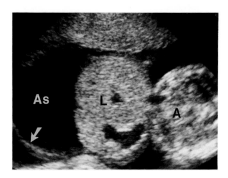

FIG. 21.7. Ascites within an omphalocele. A transverse image of the abdomen (A) at 28 weeks shows marked ascites (As) within the membrane (*arrow*) of an omphalocele. L, liver.

Limb-Body Wall Complex

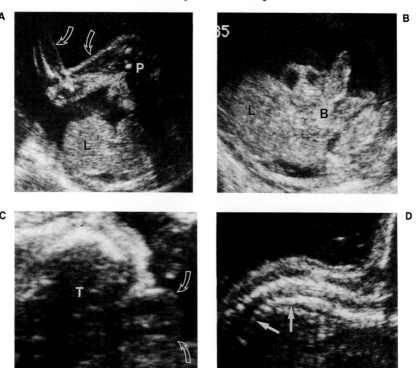

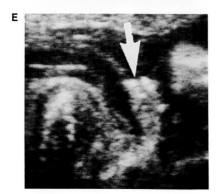

FIG. 21.8. Limb-body wall complex. **A:** An image at 18 weeks shows the lower extremity (*arrows*), pelvis (P), and eviscerated liver (L) but not the abdomen, which is outside the imaging plane because of scoliosis. **B:** An image of the same fetus shows extensively eviscerated liver (L) and bowel (B). **C:** A transverse image of the thorax (T) of the same fetus shows the cardiac ventricles (*arrows*) extending through a thoracic defect (ectopia cordia). (From ref. 1, with permission.) **D:** An image of the spine of the same fetus shows associated scoliosis (*arrows*). **E:** An image of an upper extremity of the same fetus shows a marked reduction abnormality (*arrow*). (From ref. 2, with permission.)

Limb-Body Wall Complex (*contd.*)

As a result of abnormal formation of the chorion and amnion, abdominal and possibly thoracic contents are extensively eviscerated through a large body wall defect, and the umbilical cord is abnormally confined by membranes that are closely associated with the placenta. Multiple additional anomalies are likely to be present, including scoliosis, limb defects, craniofacial defects, and neural tube defects. This combination of anomalies is lethal.

Single Umbilical Artery

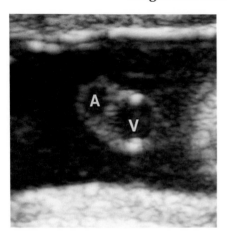

FIG. 21.9. Single umbilical artery. A transverse image of the umbilical cord at 34 weeks shows a larger umbilical vein (V) and a smaller single umbilical artery (A).

The umbilical cord contains only two vessels rather than the usual three because of the absence of one of the two arteries that normally accompany the vein. This finding is associated with an increased likelihood of other anomalies and chromosomal abnormalities.

Other Umbilical Cord Abnormalities

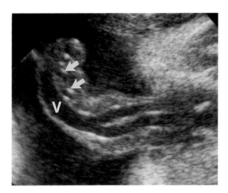

FIG. 21.10. Branching umbilical vein. A longitudinal image of the umbilical cord at 30 weeks shows abnormal branching of the umbilical vein (V) in a fetus with trisomy 18. *Arrows*, umbilical arteries.

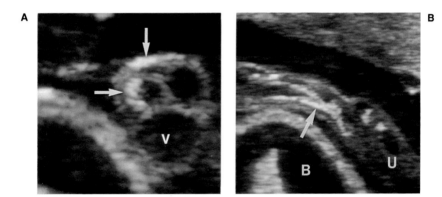

FIG. 21.11. Calcification of the umbilical cord. **A:** A transverse image of the umbilical cord at 36 weeks in a fetus with gastroschisis shows calcifications (*arrows*), presumably related to inflammation. V, vein. **B:** A longitudinal image of the same umbilical cord (U) shows extensive calcification (*arrow*) along the vessel margins as well as adjacent dilated thick-walled herniated bowel (B).

References

1. Hegge FN, Lees MH, Watson PT. Utility of a screening examination of the fetal cardiac position and four chambers during obstetric sonography. *J Reprod Med* 1987;32:353–8.
2. Hegge FN, Prescott GH, Watson PT. Utility of a screening examination of the fetal extremities during obstetrical sonography. *J Ultrasound Med* 1986; 5:639–45.

Chapter 22

THE URINARY BLADDER

Outlet Obstruction

A

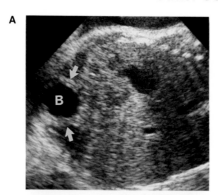

B

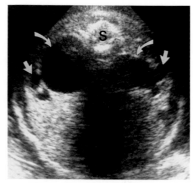

C

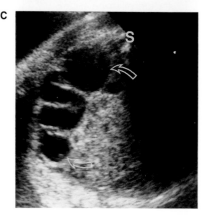

FIG. 22.1. Thickened bladder wall with posterior urethral valves. **A:** A coronal image of the abdomen of a male fetus at 36 weeks shows a thickened bladder wall (*arrows*) but a normal-sized bladder (B) in association with posterior urethral valves. **B:** A transverse image of the abdomen of the same fetus shows associated bilateral hydronephrosis, which includes pyelectasis (*curved arrows*) and caliectasis (*straight arrows*). S, spine. **C:** A transverse image of the abdomen of the same fetus shows associated hydroureter (*arrows*), which was present bilaterally. S, spine.

The urinary bladder is abnormally dilated or its wall is abnormally thickened because the outflow of urine is obstructed. This finding usually occurs in male fetuses as a result of posterior urethral valves, although other causes, such as urethral agenesis, may also occur. Associated bilateral hydroureter, hydronephrosis, or dysplastic kidneys are likely to be present,

Outlet Obstruction (*contd.*)

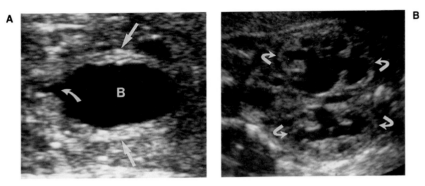

FIG. 22.2. Dilated posterior urethra with posterior urethral valves. **A:** An oblique transverse image of a male fetus at 26 weeks shows a mildly dilated urinary bladder (B) with a thickened wall (*straight arrows*) and a dilated posterior urethra (*curved arrow*) in association with posterior urethral valves. **B:** A coronal image of the abdomen of the same fetus shows associated bilateral hydronephrosis (*arrows*). Bilateral hydroureter was present as well.

and oligohydramnios may be present in severe cases. Urinoma formation from rupture of the collecting system or urine ascites from rupture or leakage from the bladder may be present as well. The abdomen may be markedly distended as a result of bladder dilatation or urine ascites.

Outlet Obstruction (*contd.*)

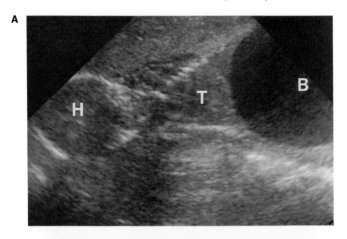

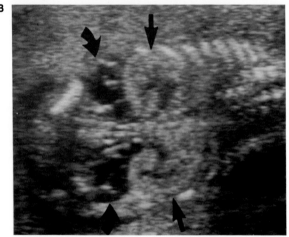

FIG. 22.3. Markedly dilated bladder with posterior urethral valves. **A:** A coronal image of a male fetus at 20 weeks shows a markedly dilated bladder (B) as well as marked oligohydramnios in association with posterior urethral valves. H, head; T, thorax. **B:** A coronal image of a similar fetus at 21 weeks shows bilateral dysplastic kidneys (*straight arrows*) and bilateral hydroureter (*curved arrows*) but very little hydronephrosis.

Outlet Obstruction (*contd.*)

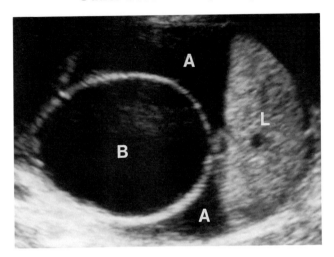

FIG. 22.4. Urine ascites with posterior urethral valves. A coronal image of the abdomen of a male fetus at 29 weeks shows a dilated bladder (B) and urine ascites (A) in association with posterior urethral valves. L, liver.

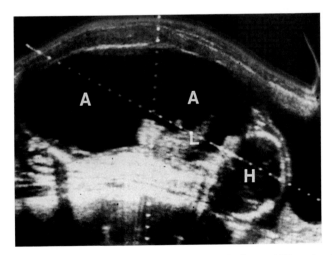

FIG. 22.5. Extreme urine ascites. A sagittal image of a fetus at 27 weeks shows extreme ascites (A), which has deformed the chest so that the entire uterus is filled by the markedly distended abdomen together with the head (H). L, liver.

Outlet Obstruction (*contd.*)

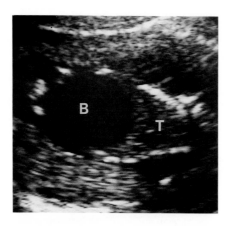

FIG. 22.6. Urethral agenesis. A coronal image of the thorax (T) and abdomen at 13 weeks shows a markedly dilated bladder (B) found to be secondary to urethral agenesis in a female fetus.

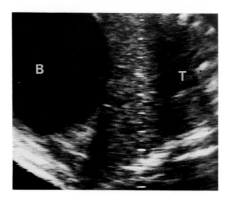

FIG. 22.7. Dilated bladder from maternal medication. A coronal image of the thorax (T) and abdomen at 39 weeks in a female fetus shows a dilated bladder (B) found to be secondary to medication to prevent spasm of the maternal bladder.

Ectopic Ureterocele

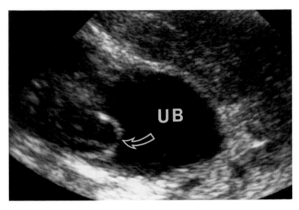

FIG. 22.8. Ectopic ureterocele. An image of the bladder (UB) at 38 weeks shows an internal thin-walled cyst (*arrow*) in association with duplication of a renal collecting system.

In association with duplication of the renal collecting system, a thin-walled cyst is present within the urinary bladder at the site of entry of a duplicated ureter.

Persistent Empty Bladder and Oligohydramnios

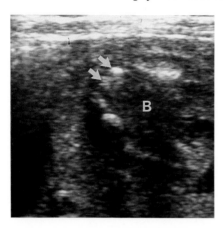

FIG. 22.9. Nonvisualization of the bladder with bilateral renal agenesis. A transverse image of the pelvis at 23 weeks at the level of the sacrum (*arrows*) and iliac wings shows persistent nonvisualization of fluid in the region of the bladder (B) and marked oligohydramnios. Fetal kidneys also could not be visualized.

A persistently empty urinary bladder together with profound oligohydramnios usually indicates bilaterally absent renal function, such as with bilateral renal agenesis or bilateral multicystic kidneys. Associated renal absence or renal abnormalities are usually identifiable as well and help to exclude the alternate possibilities of severe intrauterine growth retardation or ruptured membranes.

Urinary Bladder Exstrophy

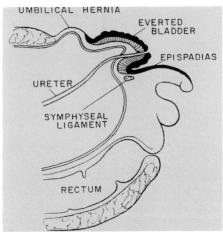

FIG. 22.10. Bladder exstrophy. A drawing shows an everted bladder and a ureter emptying outside of the body, abnormalities that account for the expected sonographic findings of a suprapubic mass, a normal amniotic fluid volume, and no visualized fluid in the bladder. (From ref. 1, with permission.)

A defect is present through the lower abdominal wall and the anterior wall of the urinary bladder, which causes the urinary bladder to be everted through the abdominal wall. Urinary bladder filling does not occur because the urinary bladder opens into the amniotic fluid. However, oligohydramnios does not occur, as with bilateral renal agenesis or multicystic kidneys, because the unobstructed ureters may empty directly into the amniotic fluid. Also, a mass that represents the everted urinary bladder may be visualized.

Cloacal Exstrophy

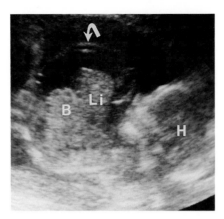

FIG. 22.11. Cloacal exstrophy. A sagittal image of a fetus at 17 weeks shows a complex omphalocele (*arrow*) containing liver (Li) and bowel (B), nonvisualization of the sacrum, and nonvisualization of the bladder in association with cloacal exstrophy. H, head. Oligohydramnios is not apparent despite associated urinary tract obstruction because the fetus was one of a pair of monoamniotic twins.

A defect is present through the lower abdominal wall, through the anterior and posterior wall of the urinary bladder, and through the anterior wall of the bowel, which causes the contiguous bowel and split halves of the urinary bladder to be everted through the body wall. A complex body wall defect may include evisceration of other abdominal organs as well. Consequently, there may be no visualized filling of the urinary bladder together with a complex body wall defect.

Reference

1. Muecke EC. In: Walsh PC, ed. *Campbell's urology*, 5th ed. Philadelphia: WB Saunders, 1986;1856–80.

Chapter 23

THE EXTREMITIES

Marked Micromelia with Lethal Dwarfism

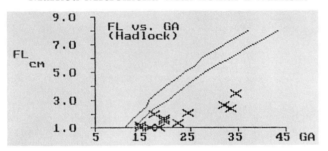

FIG. 23.1. Marked micromelia with lethal dwarfism. A graph of femur length (FL) versus gestational age (GA) for 12 measurements in 11 fetuses with lethal dwarfism shows that femur lengths are clearly abnormal by the early second trimester and markedly abnormal by the late second trimester.

Lethal dwarfism includes a somewhat diverse group of skeletal dysplasias that have in common lethal outcomes and generalized marked micromelia (markedly short limbs). The marked micromelia is likely to be apparent by the early second trimester and is usually obvious from imaging alone before measurements are obtained. In contrast the milder micromelia of nonlethal dwarfism is usually not apparent until later in the gestation and even then may not be immediately obvious without measurements.

Additional features are helpful in identifying the specific varieties of lethal dwarfism. Incomplete mineralization of the skull may be present with osteogenesis imperfecta type II, achondrogenesis, and hypophosphatasia. Incomplete mineralization of the spine may be present with achondrogenesis and hypophosphatasia. Multiple fractures may be present with osteogenesis imperfecta type II. Marked narrowing to the thorax is present with thanatophoric dwarfism and homozygous achondroplasia and may be present with achondrogenesis. A cloverleaf skull may be present with thanatophoric dwarfism.

Marked Micromelia with Lethal Dwarfism (*contd.*)

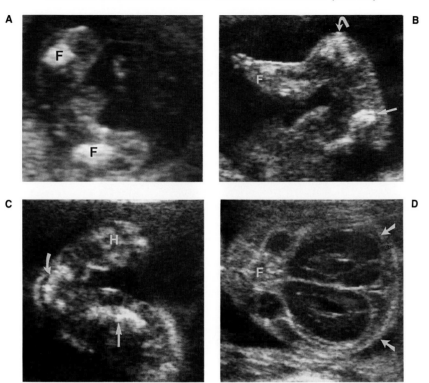

FIG. 23.2. Osteogenesis imperfecta type II. **A:** An image of the lower extremities at 16 weeks shows markedly short femurs (F). **B:** An image of a lower extremity at 19 weeks shows a markedly short femur (*straight arrow*) and a fracture of the tibia (*curved arrow*). F, foot. **C:** An image of an upper extremity at 19 weeks shows a serpiginous appearance of the humerus (*straight arrow*) and bones of the forearm (*curved arrow*) because of many fractures. H, hand. **D:** An oblique image of the anterior skull at 19 weeks shows incomplete mineralization of the cranium (*arrows*) and facial bones (F).

Marked Micromelia with Lethal Dwarfism (*contd.*)

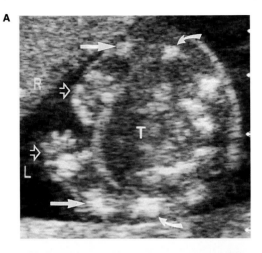

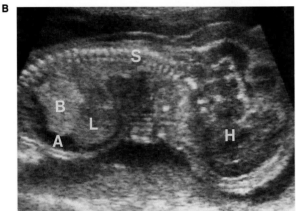

FIG. 23.3. Osteogenesis imperfecta type II. **A:** A transverse image of the thorax (T) that includes the upper extremities at 19 weeks shows markedly short humeri (*curved arrows*) and ulnae and radii (*straight arrows*). *Open arrows,* hands; R, right; L, left. **B:** A sagittal image of the same fetus shows incomplete mineralization of the skull and mild ascites (A). H, head; S, spine; L, liver; B, bowel. Follow-up was limited to clinical and radiographic examination.

Marked Micromelia with Lethal Dwarfism (*contd.*)

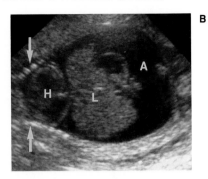

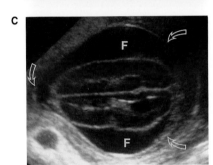

FIG. 23.4. Achondrogenesis. **A:** An image of a lower extremity at 27 weeks shows the femur (F) and tibia and fibula (TF) to be poorly defined and markedly short. **B:** A coronal image of the body of the same fetus shows a small thorax (*arrows*) as well as ascites (A) and cardiomegaly (H) from generalized hydrops. L, liver. **C:** A transverse image of the head of the same fetus shows incomplete mineralization of the cranium (*arrows*) and suspension of the brain within considerable extraaxial fluid (F) from hydrops.

Marked Micromelia with Lethal Dwarfism (*contd.*)

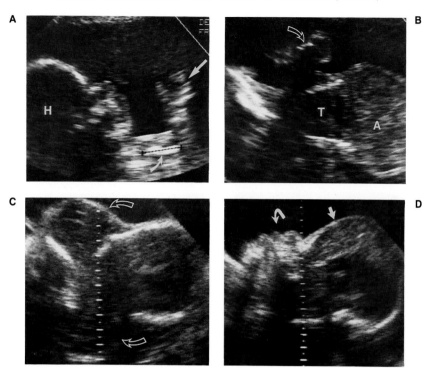

FIG. 23.5. Thanatophoric dwarfism. **A:** An image of an upper extremity at 25 weeks shows that it is markedly short compared to the size of the head (H). *Curved arrow*, humerus; *straight arrow*, hand. **B:** A coronal image of the thorax (T) and abdomen (A) of the same fetus shows narrowing of the thorax. *Arrow*, upper extremity. **C:** A coronal image of the head of a different fetus at 25 weeks shows the bitemporal prominences (*arrows*) of an associated cloverleaf skull. **D:** A sagittal image of the head of the same fetus shows an associated prominent forehead (*straight arrow*) and abnormal facial profile (*curved arrow*). (D, from ref. 1, with permission.)

Marked Micromelia with Lethal Dwarfism (*contd.*)

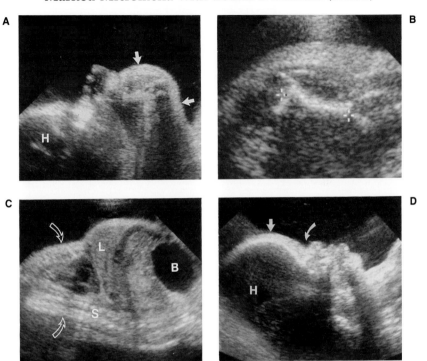

FIG. 23.6. Homozygous achondroplasia. **A:** An image of an upper extremity (*arrows*) at 34 weeks shows that it is markedly short. H, head. **B:** An image of a femur (*graticules*) of the same fetus shows that it is markedly short. **C:** An image of the trunk of the same fetus shows that the thorax (*arrows*) is abnormally small compared to the abdomen. S, spine; L, liver; B, bladder. **D:** An anterior sagittal image of the head (H) of the same fetus shows a depressed nasal bridge (*curved arrow*) and a prominent forehead (*straight arrow*) in association with moderate macrocephaly.

Nonlethal Dwarfism

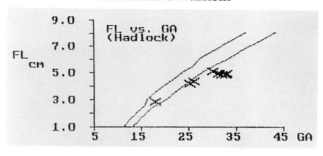

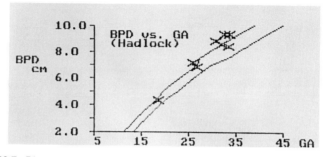

FIG. 23.7. Biometry of heterozygous (nonlethal) achondroplasia. **A:** A graph of femur length (FL) versus gestational age (GA) for eight measurements in four fetuses shows that femur lengths are normal early in the second trimester and do not become clearly abnormal until late in the second trimester. **B:** A graph of biparietal diameter (BPD) versus gestational age (GA) for eight measurements in four fetuses shows a tendency toward mild macrocephaly in the third trimester.

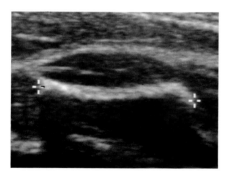

FIG. 23.8. Heterozygous achondroplasia. An image of the femur (*graticules*) at 33 weeks is not strikingly abnormal subjectively, although the measured length is abnormally short. (This femur may be compared to the femur of Fig. 23.6B.)

Micromelia with nonlethal dwarfism usually occurs later in the gestation and is of lesser magnitude than that with lethal dwarfism. In the best known variety of nonlethal dwarfism, heterozygous achondroplasia, the femur length remains within the normal range until near the end of the second trimester.

Reduction Abnormality

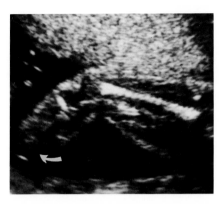

FIG. 23.9. Amputation from amniotic band syndrome. An image of a lower extremity at 28 weeks shows amputation of the foot and ankle at the level of the midcalf (*arrow*) in a fetus that also had clubfoot of the other lower extremity, asymmetric hydrocephalus, and a severe facial cleft. (From ref. 2, with permission.)

A limb or a portion of a limb is absent. Partial limb loss may occur distally or within a limb. An example of distal limb loss is amputation from amniotic band syndrome. Examples of partial loss within a limb include absence of the radius with radial aplasia and absent long bones between the hands and shoulders or between the feet and hips with phocomelia.

Reduction Abnormality (*contd.*)

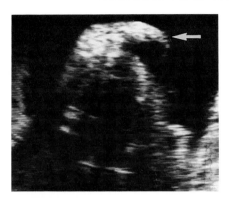

FIG. 23.10. Phocomelia. An image of an upper extremity at 27 weeks shows the hand (*arrow*) originating at the shoulder because of absence of the long bones. Similar abnormalities were present for all extremities. (From ref. 2, with permission.)

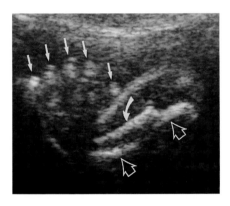

FIG. 23.11. Radial hypoplasia. An image of an upper extremity at 22 weeks shows a markedly short radius (*curved arrow*) compared to the ulna (*open arrows*) and the hand arising at a right angle from the forearm in a fetus with VATERS syndrome. *Small arrows,* digits.

Reduction Abnormality (*contd.*)

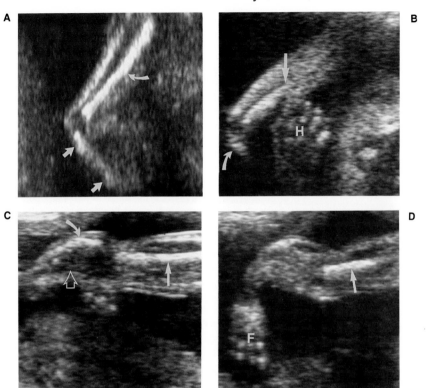

FIG. 23.12. Radial and tibial aplasia. **A:** An image of an upper extremity at 22 weeks shows a short ulna (*straight arrows*) compared to the humerus (*curved arrow*) and no visualized radius. **B:** An image of the same upper extremity shows the hand (H), which forms a right angle with the partially shown ulna (*curved arrow*), positioned near the humerus (*straight arrow*). **C:** An image of a lower extremity of the same fetus shows a short fibula (*curved arrow*) compared to the femur (*straight arrow*) and no visualized tibia (*open arrow*). **D:** An image of the same lower extremity shows the foot (F) arising at a markedly abnormal angle. *Straight arrow*, femur. There was a family history of VATERS syndrome.

Clubfoot

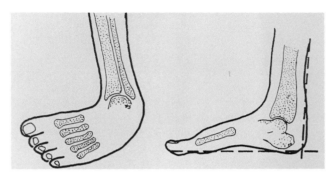

FIG. 23.13. Clubfoot compared to a normal foot. **Left:** The medial deviation and fixed plantar flexion of clubfoot, which results in the presence of the tibia, fibula, all metatarsals, and all digits in the same plane. **Right:** A normal foot with only the tibia, one metatarsal, and one digit in the same plane. (From ref. 3, with permission.)

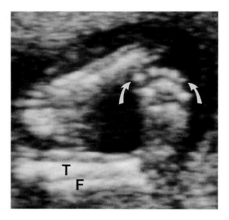

FIG. 23.14. Clubfoot. An image of a lower extremity at 18 weeks shows the tibia (T), fibula (F), all digits (*arrows*), and all metatarsal heads in the same imaging plane.

Fixed plantar flexion and medial deviation of the foot is present. As a result all of the metatarsals and toes are aligned medially in the same plane with both the tibia and the fibula.

Polydactyly, Syndactyly, and Clinodactyly

A
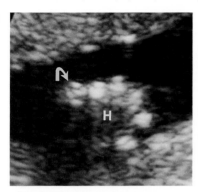

B
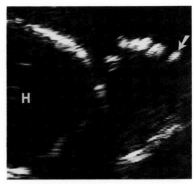

FIG. 23.15. Polydactyly. **A:** An image through the digits of the hand (H) at 17 weeks shows a sixth digit (*arrow*) on the ulnar side in a fetus with Meckel-Gruber syndrome. **B:** An image through the digits of the hand at 21 weeks shows a sixth digit (*arrow*) on the ulnar side in a fetus with chondroectodermal dysplasia. H, head. (B, from ref. 2, with permission.)

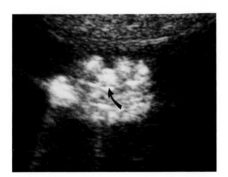

FIG. 23.16. Clinodactyly. An image through the digits of the hand at 32 weeks shows persistent overlapping of one digit (*arrow*) in a fetus with trisomy 18.

With polydactyly extra digits are present; with syndactyly fused digits are present; and with clinodactyly fixed deviation of digits is present. Polydactyly may occur with other anomalies as a part of several syndromes, such as trisomy 13 and Meckel-Gruber syndrome. Syndactyly and clinodactyly may also occur with other anomalies and with chromosomal abnormalities.

Fractures

Fractures of long bones and ribs may be present with osteogenesis imperfecta and possibly with hypophosphatasia as discussed under lethal dwarfism.

Abnormal Muscle

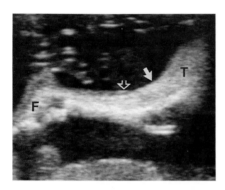

FIG. 23.17. Reduced muscle mass with contracture. An image of a lower extremity at 24 weeks shows markedly reduced soft tissue in the region of the gastrocnemius muscle (*open arrow*) and absence of the popliteal crease (*closed arrow*) in a fetus with sacral agenesis. T, thigh; F, foot.

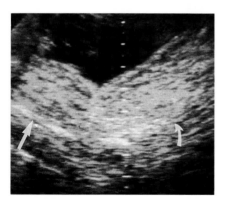

FIG. 23.18. Hyperechoic muscle with spinal cord disease. An image of a lower extremity at 31 weeks shows degenerating muscle so hyperechoic that the bone cannot be separately defined in a fetus with spinal muscular atrophy. *Curved arrow*, thigh; *straight arrow*, calf. (From ref. 2, with permission.)

Muscle volume may be decreased, muscle echogenicity may be increased, and soft tissue contour may be abnormal in association with contractures or abnormal innervation.

Subcutaneous Edema

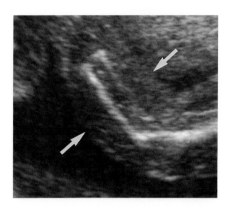

FIG. 23.19. Extremity subcutaneous edema with cystic hygroma. An image of a lower extremity at 22 weeks shows marked thickening of the subcutaneous region (*arrows*) in association with a posterior cystic hygroma and generalized lymphedema.

The subcutaneous tissue of the extremities is abnormally thickened because of edema from hydrops with congestive heart failure or from lymphedema with cystic hygroma and generalized lymphedema.

References

1. Hegge FN, Prescott GH, Watson PT. Fetal facial abnormalities identified during obstetric sonography. *J Ultrasound Med* 1986;5:679–84.
2. Hegge FN, Prescott GH, Watson PT. Utility of a screening examination of the fetal extremities during obstetrical sonography. *J Ultrasound Med* 1986;5:639–45.
3. Jeanty P, Romero R, d'Alton M, Ingeborg V, Hobbins JC. In utero sonographic detection of hand and foot deformities. *J Ultrasound Med* 1985;4:595–601.

Chapter 24

ANOMALIES ASSOCIATED WITH MULTIPLE GESTATIONS

Monoamniotic Twins

A small percentage of identical (monozygotic) twins are present within one amniotic sac rather than within separate sacs. An interamniotic membrane is consequently not present, and entanglement of the umbilical cords is likely. The twins are ordinarily delivered early to prevent the known late third trimester high mortality from umbilical cord entanglement.

Monoamniotic Twins (*contd.*)

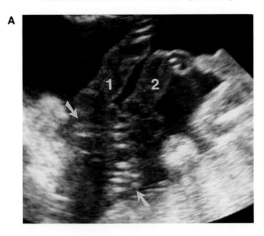

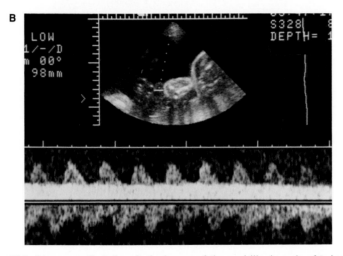

Fig. 24.1. Monozygotic twins. **A:** An image of the umbilical cords of twins (1,2) shows both cords extending into a region of entanglement (*arrows*). **B:** A pulse Doppler image confirms the presence of both umbilical cords in the region of entanglement by showing two differing umbilical arterial signals that are out of phase with each other. A separating interamniotic membrane was not visualized.

Twin-Twin Transfusion

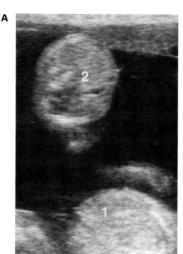

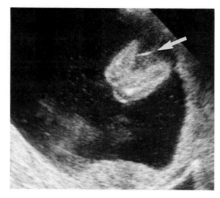

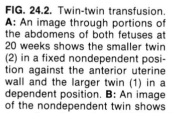

FIG. 24.2. Twin-twin transfusion.
A: An image through portions of
the abdomens of both fetuses at
20 weeks shows the smaller twin
(2) in a fixed nondependent position against the anterior uterine
wall and the larger twin (1) in a
dependent position. **B:** An image
of the nondependent twin shows
a small portion of amniotic membrane (*arrow*) that was difficult to visualize,
consistent with the stuck twin appearance caused by polyhydramnios of the 1
sac and oligohydramnios of the 2 sac. **C:** A transverse image of both twins at 25
weeks (after therapeutic amniocentesis of the 1 sac) shows markedly discordant
size of the two abdomens and ascites (A) of the 1 abdomen from early hydrops.

In identical twins with a single placenta, abnormal arterial to venous
anastomoses between the two circulations may result in significant
shunting of blood from one twin to the other. Initially, growth retardation
and oligohydramnios occur with the donor twin, and increased size and
polyhydramnios occur with the recipient twin. This is one cause of the
"stuck twin" syndrome, in which the interamniotic membrane is closely
applied to the smaller twin, which remains confined to a fixed, possibly
nondependent position against the uterine wall. If untreated, this syndrome often leads to hydrops of the recipient twin and death of both twins.

Acardiac Twin (Reversed Arterial Perfusion Sequence)

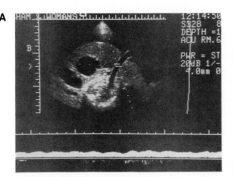

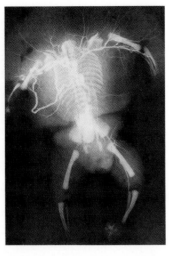

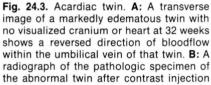

Fig. 24.3. Acardiac twin. **A:** A transverse image of a markedly edematous twin with no visualized cranium or heart at 32 weeks shows a reversed direction of bloodflow within the umbilical vein of that twin. **B:** A radiograph of the pathologic specimen of the abnormal twin after contrast injection shows absence of a normal heart as well as absence of the head and portions of the upper extremities. (From ref. 1, copyright © 1989 by John Wiley & Sons, Inc. Reprinted by permission of John Wiley & Sons, Inc.)

In identical twins with a single placenta, abnormal arterial-to-arterial and venous-to-venous anastomosis between the two circulations may result in abnormal perfusion of one twin by the other by way of reversed flow in the arteries and veins of the perfused twin. Many anomalies are present in the perfused twin, particularly in the upper body and head, where perfusion is poorest with this sequence. Consequently, the most striking anomalies in the perfused twin may include absence or marked deformity of the head and upper extremities and absence of a pulsatile heart. The other twin may develop cardiomegaly and hydrops.

Conjoined Twins

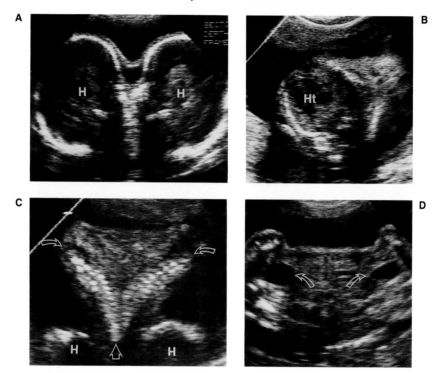

Fig. 24.4. Conjoined twins **A:** An image of the heads (H) at 25 weeks shows partial fusion near the bases of the skulls. **B:** A transverse image of the same fetus shows a fused thorax, which contains a single heart (Ht). **C:** A coronal image of the same fetus shows two spines (*curved arrows*) that diverge from a fused cervical region (*straight arrow*). H, head. **D:** A transverse image of the same fetus shows two pelves diverging from the fused thoracoabdominal region. *Arrows*, urinary bladders.

Identical twins are partly fused because of incomplete separation early in development. The fusion may occur at any level from the head to the sacrum but most commonly involves the thorax or abdomen. Many configurations of conjoined twins are consequently possible.

Concordant Anomalies

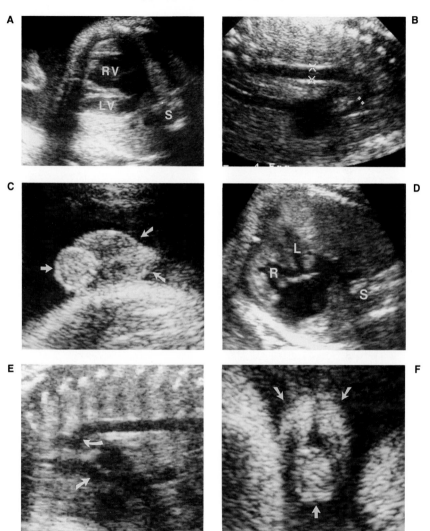

Fig. 24.5. Concordant anomalies in monozygotic twins. **Twin 1: A:** A transverse image of the thorax at 28 weeks shows a hypoplastic left ventricle (LV) and a large right ventricle (RV). S, spine. **B:** A parasagittal image of the aorta shows a hypoplastic arch (*graticules*) compared to the descending portion (*graticules*). **C:** An image near the perineum shows ambiguous genitalia (*arrows*). **Twin 2: D:** A transverse image of the thorax at 28 weeks shows a hypoplastic left ventricle (L) and a large right ventricle (R). S, spine. **E:** A parasagittal image of the aorta shows a poorly defined arch between the proximal (*straight arrow*) and distal (*curved arrow*) portions, which was shown to be hypoplastic on follow-up examinations. **F:** An image near the perineum shows ambiguous genitalia (*arrows*).

Concordant Anomalies (*contd.*)

The likelihood of anomalies is somewhat increased in twins, particularly in identical twins. Usually anomalies are limited to one of the two fetuses. In identical twins, however, anomalies are occasionally concordant in the two fetuses.

Reference

1. Benson CB, Bieber FR, Genest DR, Doubilet PM. Doppler demonstration of reversed umbilical blood flow in an acardiac twin. *J Clin Ultrasound* 1989;17:291–5.

Chapter 25

ANOMALIES ASSOCIATED WITH CHROMOSOMAL ABNORMALITIES

Turner's Syndrome

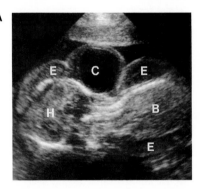
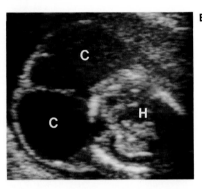

FIG. 25.1. Turner's syndrome. **A:** Posterior cystic hygroma (C) and extensive subcutaneous lymphedema (E) surrounding the head (H) and body (B) at 17 weeks. **B:** Bilocular cystic hygroma (C) posterior to the head (H) at 13 weeks. **C:** Bilateral pleural effusions (F) and thoracic subcutaneous lymphedema (E) at 21 weeks. **D:** Ascites (F) surrounding liver (L) at 19 weeks. **E:** Abdominal subcutaneous lymphedema (E) at 17 weeks. **F:** Hypoplastic left ventricle (LV) and large right ventricle (RV) at 19 weeks. **G:** Bilateral cystic dysplastic kidneys (*arrows*) and ascites (A) at 19 weeks. (*Figure continues next page.*)

Turner's syndrome (45,X) is commonly associated with a posterior cystic hygroma and generalized lymphedema, although these abnormalities may also occur with other chromosomal abnormalities or with normal chromosomes. Cardiac anomalies, particularly of the left side, and urinary tract anomalies are also more frequent with Turner's syndrome. Fetuses with a posterior cystic hygroma and generalized lymphedema in association with Turner's syndrome are likely to die *in utero*. Other fetuses with Turner's syndrome may survive with variable disability.

Turner's Syndrome (*contd.*)

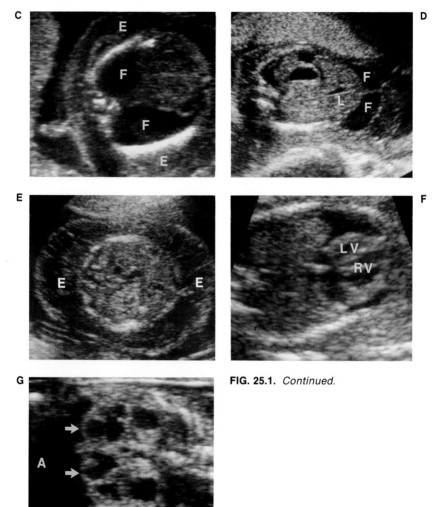

FIG. 25.1. *Continued.*

Triploidy

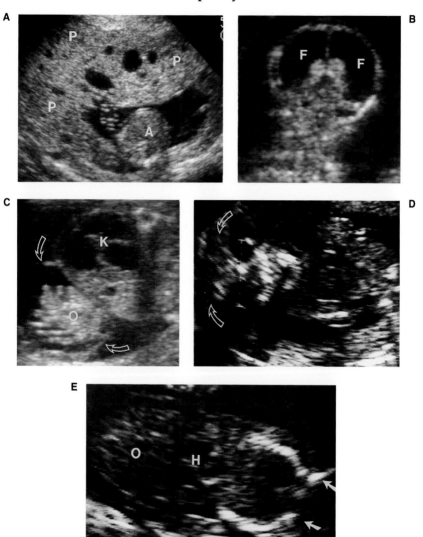

FIG. 25.2. Triploidy. **A:** Multicystic placenta (P), which is markedly enlarged compared to the fetal abdomen (A) at 13 weeks. **B:** Abnormal intracranial fluid (F) in the same fetus. **C:** Omphalocele (O) with a surrounding membrane (*arrows*) and a multicystic kidney (K) in a different fetus at 21 weeks. **D:** Anencephaly (*arrows superior to the orbits and facial bones*) in a different fetus at 16 weeks. **E:** Marked spinal dysraphism (*arrows*), ectopia cordis (H), and omphalocele (O) in the same fetus as shown in D.

Triploidy (*contd.*)

Triploidy may be associated with numerous anomalies of many organ systems. Multiple anomalies may be present in the same fetus. In addition severe growth retardation of the fetus is present, and the placenta is likely to be thickened and multicystic (partial molar placenta). Fetuses with triploidy do not survive.

Trisomy 21

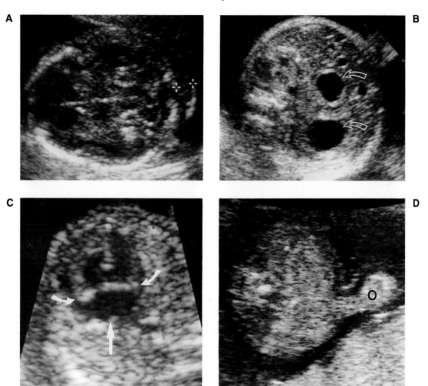

FIG. 25.3. Trisomy 21. **A:** Posterior nuchal thickening at 18 weeks. **B:** Duodenal atresia causing a double bubble (*arrows*) at 30 weeks. **C:** Atrioventricular canal with characteristic common valvular (*curved arrows*) and septal (*straight arrow*) abnormalities at 18 weeks. **D:** Omphalocele (O) at 17 weeks.

Trisomy 21 is occasionally associated with some anomalies such as duodenal atresia, atrioventricular canal, cystic hygroma, omphalocele, and posterior nuchal thickening, but well-defined sonographic anomalies are usually not present. Also, fetuses with mildly short femur lengths may have a somewhat increased likelihood of trisomy 21 (1). The use of this finding to identify subjects for genetic amniocentesis is controversial and must be validated in any laboratory where it is done. Fetuses with trisomy 21 are likely to survive with variable disability.

Trisomy 18

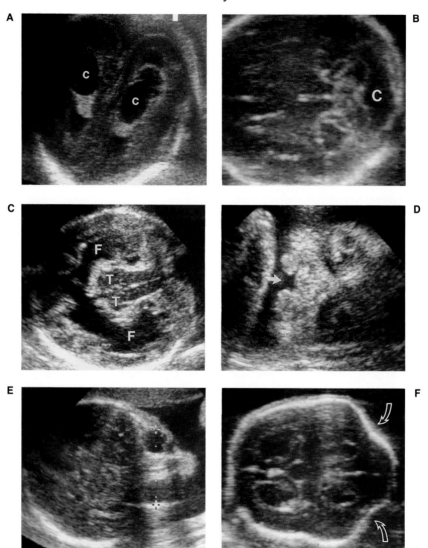

FIG. 25.4. Trisomy 18—head and neck. **A:** Bilateral large choroid plexus cysts (C) at 19 weeks. **B:** Large cisterna magna (C) at 26 weeks. **C:** Holoprosencephaly with monoventricular system (F) and fused thalami (T) at 35 weeks. **D:** Median facial cleft (*arrow*) with holoprosencephaly shown previously. **E:** Hypotelorism (*graticules*) at 33 weeks. **F:** Lemon sign (*arrows*) with spina bifida at 23 weeks.

Trisomy 18 (*contd.*)

G

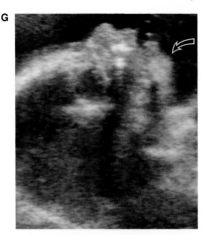

G: Abnormal facial profile with mild micrognathia (*arrow*) at 31 weeks.

Trisomy 18 may be associated with a single umbilical artery and with numerous anomalies of all organ systems, particularly cardiovascular anomalies and anomalies of the hands and feet. Fetuses with trisomy 18 are likely to die soon after birth, although some may survive somewhat longer with severe disability. Most fetuses with trisomy 18 found to be abnormal by ultrasound at Emanuel Hospital have had multiple anomalies. In the accompanying figures, examples of those anomalies are shown individually without listing the particular combinations found in each fetus.

Trisomy 18 (*contd.*)

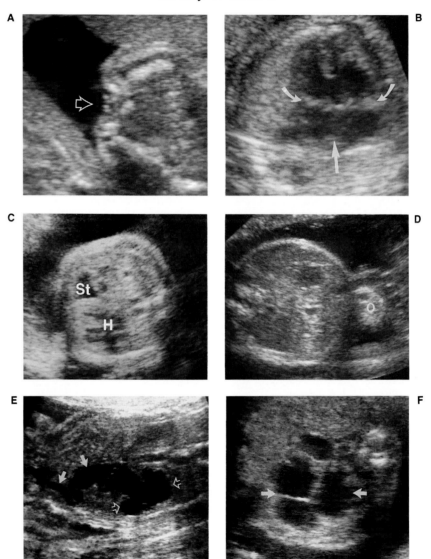

FIG. 25.5. Trisomy 18—thorax and abdomen. **A:** Open spina bifida (*arrow*) at 23 weeks. **B:** Atrioventricular canal with common valvular (*curved arrows*) and septal (*straight arrow*) abnormalities at 26 weeks. **C:** Diaphragmatic hernia with the stomach (St) in the left thorax and the heart (H) in the right thorax at 34 weeks. **D:** Omphalocele (O) at 32 weeks. **E:** Upper pole hydronephrotic sac (*open arrows*) and hydroureter (*closed arrows*) with a duplex kidney at 35 weeks. **F:** Multicystic kidney (*arrows*) at 22 weeks.

Trisomy 18 (*contd.*)

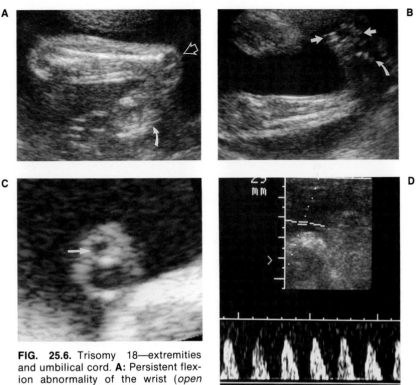

FIG. 25.6. Trisomy 18—extremities and umbilical cord. **A:** Persistent flexion abnormality of the wrist (*open arrow*) at 26 weeks. *Curved arrow*, hand. **B:** Clubfoot at 26 weeks. *Straight arrows*, toes; *curved arrow*, metatarsals. **C:** Single umbilical artery (*straight arrow*) at 34 weeks. **D:** Umbilical artery waveform showing reversed diastolic flow at 36 weeks.

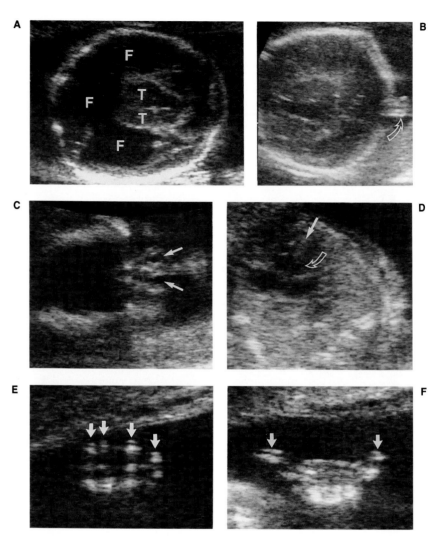

FIG. 25.7. Trisomy 13—anomalous 16-week fetus. **A:** Holoprosencephaly with monoventricular hydrocephalus (F) surrounding fused thalami (T). **B:** Proboscis (*arrow*). **C:** Small eyes with extreme hypotelorism (*arrows*) compatible with cyclopia. **D:** Cardiac ventricular septal defect (*curved arrow*). *Straight arrow*, ventricular septum. **E:** Polydactyly. Four fingers (*arrows*). **F:** Polydactyly. Thumb and sixth finger (*arrows*).

Trisomy 13 may be associated with a single umbilical artery and with numerous anomalies of all organ systems, particularly holoprosencephaly, associated facial anomalies, cardiovascular anomalies, and anomalies of

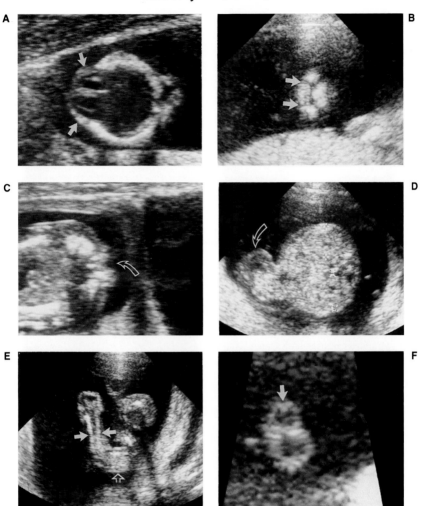

FIG. 25.8. Trisomy 13—anomalous 17-week fetus. **A:** Encephalocele (*arrows*). **B:** Abnormal face (*arrows*). **C:** Open spina bifida (*arrow*). **D:** Omphalocele (*arrow*). **E:** Clubfoot (*open arrow*) in same plane as the tibia and fibula (*closed arrows*). **F:** Single umbilical artery (*arrow*).

the hands and feet, such as polydactyly and clubfoot. Multiple anomalies may be present in the same fetus. Fetuses with trisomy 13 are likely to die soon after birth, although some may survive somewhat longer with severe impairment.

Trisomy 13 (*contd.*)

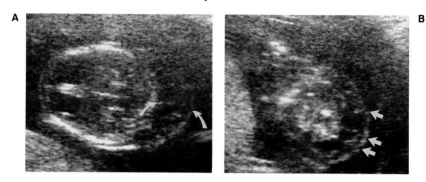

FIG. 25.9. Trisomy 13—anomalous 14-week fetus. **A:** Small posterior cystic hygroma (*arrows*) at the base of the skull. **B:** Same cystic hygroma at the level of the neck appears to show septation (*arrows*).

Reference

1. Benacerraf BR, Gelman R, Frigoletto FD Jr. Sonographic identification of second-trimester fetuses with Down's syndrome. *N Engl J Med* 1987;317:1371–6.

Subject Index